LindaRhodes
caregiving

Caregiving As Your Parents Age

Linda Rhodes
caregiving

Caregiving As Your Parents Age

DR. LINDA RHODES

Previously published as *The Complete Idiot's Guide® to Caring for Aging Parents*

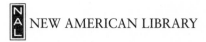 NEW AMERICAN LIBRARY

New American Library
Published by New American Library, a division of
Penguin Group (USA) Inc., 375 Hudson Street,
New York, New York 10014, USA
Penguin Group (Canada), 10 Alcorn Avenue, Toronto,
Ontario M4V 3B2, Canada (a division of Pearson Penguin Canada Inc.)
Penguin Books Ltd., 80 Strand, London WC2R 0RL, England
Penguin Ireland, 25 St. Stephen's Green, Dublin 2,
Ireland (a division of Penguin Books Ltd.)
Penguin Group (Australia), 250 Camberwell Road, Camberwell, Victoria 3124,
Australia (a division of Pearson Australia Group Pty. Ltd.)
Penguin Books India Pvt. Ltd., 11 Community Centre, Panchsheel Park,
New Delhi - 110 017, India
Penguin Group (NZ), cnr Airborne and Rosedale Roads, Albany,
Auckland 1310, New Zealand (a division of Pearson New Zealand Ltd.)
Penguin Books (South Africa) (Pty.) Ltd., 24 Sturdee Avenue,
Rosebank, Johannesburg 2196, South Africa

Penguin Books Ltd., Registered Offices:
80 Strand, London WC2R 0RL, England

Published by New American Library, a division of Penguin Group (USA) Inc. Previously published as
The Complete Idiot's Guide® to Caring for Aging Parents. Also previously published in an Alpha edition.

First New American Library Printing, March 2005
10 9 8 7 6 5 4 3 2 1

Library of Congress Catalog Card Number: 2003103304

Printed in the United States of America

PUBLISHER'S NOTE
Every effort has been made to ensure that the information contained in this book is complete and accurate. However
neither the publisher nor the author is engaged in rendering professional advice or services to the individual reader.
The ideas, procedures, and suggestions contained in this book are not intended as a substitute for consulting with
your physician. All matters regarding your health require medical supervision. Neither the author nor the publisher
shall be liable or responsible for any loss or damage allegedly arising from any information or suggestion in this book.
The opinions expressed in this book represent the personal views of the author and not of the publisher.

While the author has made every effort to provide accurate telephone numbers and Internet addresses at the time
of publication, neither the publisher nor the author assumes any responsibility for errors, or for changes that occur
after publication.

To my Mom and Dad, Shirley M. Baressi and John W. Colvin.
May I do as well by you as you have by me.

Contents at a Glance

Contents

Appendixes

Foreword

As a responsible government official for many years, I am acutely aware of the great many needs of America's aged. For millions of elderly, their Social Security check is the bedrock of their retirement income. As a partner with the Medicare program, Social Security also handles retiree's enrollment for Medicare hospital benefits and doctor bills and is often able to provide direction to related federal, state, and local programs. Social Security, Medicare, and allied programs have contributed enormously to the well-being of the elderly.

One of my persistent concerns is how to best reach out to the American public, informing them of the many government benefits and services available to them. In my travels across the country, I am continually surprised to learn how little the public really understands what they are entitled to. But it's no wonder: In today's fast-paced and complex world, far too many of us are caught up in the urgency of our own lives. It's hard to find the time or energy to track down benefits and services that can help our loved ones.

And that's where Dr. Linda Rhodes' book can make a difference. *Caregiving as Your Parents Age* anticipates the many practical questions you may have in taking care of your parents. Whether they live with you, across town, or thousands of miles away, Dr. Rhodes shows you how to stay on top of your parents' health care, how to navigate the world of geriatric care, and where to track down community services. One special feature of the book is her Nursing Home Navigator, a guide that helps you find a high-quality nursing home worthy of your parents.

The book is easy to use and an excellent reference to Web sites that will save you hours in finding a wide range of resources to help you care for your parents. And Dr. Rhodes knows your needs and challenges because she's lived them: Not only does she have extensive professional experience as Pennsylvania's former Secretary of Aging, and as a long-time advocate for the aging, she has the real-life experience of caring in her own home for an older family member who suffered from a stroke and dementia.

Do your parents a great favor and read this book. I wish I had this book available during the years I was taking care of my recently departed mother. Whether you have an immediate problem to solve or just want to assure you are not missing something you should know or be doing, this book can help you.

—Stanford G. Ross, former U.S. Commissioner of the Social Security Administration and Public Trustee of the Social Security and Medicare Trust Funds

Introduction

During my years as Secretary of Aging for the state of Pennsylvania, I received countless questions from baby boomer friends about what they should do for their parents. How do I get my dad to a good geriatrician? How do I *find* a geriatrician? Who can I call to figure out whether or not my mom has Alzheimer's? How do I know it's safe for my mom to live alone? What's the deal with Medi-gap insurance? Are Medicare managed care plans a safe bet? How do you find a good nursing home?

I figure my friends aren't so different from the rest of the world. And so the seeds for this book were sown.

So many people today are under the misconception that Americans automatically place their aging parents in nursing homes. Nothing could be further from the truth. A mere fraction—less than 5 percent—of the elderly live in a long-term care facility. Residents are there because they are very sick; rarely is it because they have been abandoned by their family. Every day, daughters, sons, and spouses are making quiet, often heroic, efforts to care for their aging loved ones. This book is for them.

How to Use This Book

Caregiving As Your Parents Age is divided into five parts. The book begins with an overview of the process of aging. **Part 1, "Seeing Aging Through Your Parents' Eyes,"** explores aging in American culture and then takes you through the major physical changes everyone experiences. Each chapter then progresses to more common physical and mental problems that many people face as they age. This part concludes with the basics on the "big four" that many people fear: cancer, heart attacks, strokes, and Alzheimer's.

Once you have a solid understanding of the mental and physical aspects of aging, **Part 2, "The World of Geriatric Health Care,"** takes you through the health care system. You'll learn the world of geriatrics, what to watch for when your parent has a hospital stay, how to track down home health care, and how to stay on top of your parent's medications.

There are plenty of options available today for your parents: They can stay at home, live in the community, find a creative housing option, or opt for assisted living. Perhaps, a continuing care retirement community makes sense or it might be time to secure nursing home care. **Part 3, "Understanding You and Your Parents' Options,"** describes each living arrangement, arming you with consumer tips so you'll know what to look for and what option is the best for your parents given their set of circumstances.

If your mom or dad does come to live with you, **Part 4, "Caregiving: Coming to Live with You,"** helps you assess whether or not this is the best decision for both you and your parent. You're then given practical strategies on caring for your parent in the home, how to juggle your work with caregiving, and how to maintain your stamina. The last chapter is helpful whether or not you take care of your parents in the home. It helps you understand the benefits of hospice and advance directives, and how to have a heart-to-heart discussion with your parent about death and dying.

Part 5, "Financial and Legal Matters," navigates you through Medicare, Medicaid, and the Veterans Administration medical system. You'll learn the importance of Medi-gap insurance policies and the differences between traditional and HMO (managed care) Medicare, pick up some tips on how to beat out-of-pocket expenses, and find out what to really look for in a long-term care insurance policy. Planning for incapacity through living wills, durable power of attorney, and guardianship are issues that most of us don't like to talk about, but there's a chapter with a concise, compassionate explanation of the steps you need to take. We even guide you through the conversation with your parents. And where would we be without lawyers? There's a chapter on elder lawyers, and the basics of wills and estate planning.

We also include four helpful appendixes: Resources, National List of State Units on Aging, a Nursing Home Site Visit Guide, and a Nursing Home Bill of Rights.

Extras

In each chapter, we've included boxes that present interesting and helpful information.

A Word About Style

This book is written for the sons and daughters of aging parents. The information throughout this book, however, can be just as helpful to spouses who are also caregivers.

Rather than being too formal or too cumbersome by always referring to "your parent," you'll find that I interchange references to either your mom or dad. Of course, either reference applies to most any situation discussed in this book.

Acknowledgments

Two people who have passed on influenced this book in ways they never knew: Lena Richards, my children's great-grandmother, came to live with us for a year. I had the honor of caring for her. The *heart* in this book comes from what I learned from living with Grandma. And the late Governor Robert P. Casey of Pennsylvania for believing in me and appointing me as his Secretary of Aging. The *advocacy* in this book comes from being his partner in a grand fight for the elderly of our state.

A special thanks goes to my editor, Lynn Northrup, who not only guided the book through the tests of grammar and style but cheered me on to the finish line. Three colleagues who took time out of their busy schedules to make sure I got it right are Rose G. Ferraro, founder of the Forbes Center for Gerontology in Pittsburgh, Pennsylvania; Bernice Soffer, founder of the nationally recognized ombudsman program, CARIE; and Shelly Sommerhof Levin, Physician Liaison, Hospice of Baltimore. And for his terrific research skills, many thanks to Ed Powers, formerly with the Centers of Disease Control.

And to my husband Eric B. Schnurer, thanks for the coaching, the dinners, letting go of weekends, and always, always being there for me. Finally, Matthew and Brennan, please keep this book handy when in the not-too-distant future your dear mom needs you to read it. Thanks for being two great kids that I know I can count on.

A Special Thanks to the Technical Reviewer

Caregiving as Your Parents Age was reviewed by an expert who not only checked the accuracy of what you'll learn in this book, but also provided invaluable insight to help ensure that this book tells you everything you need to know about caring for your aging parents. Our special thanks are extended to Roger J. Cadieux, M.D.

Dr. Cadieux is a Clinical Professor of Psychiatry in the Department of Psychiatry at the Pennsylvania State University College of Medicine at Hershey and is a Fellow of the American Psychiatric Association. Dr. Cadieux is also the Physician Consultant to the Pennsylvania Department of Aging.

Dr. Cadieux has participated on the National HCFA Advisory Committee for applying drug use review to the Medicare/Medicaid population, and is an active advisor on the Commonwealth of Pennsylvania's Pharmaceutical Therapeutic Advisory Committee for the Elderly. Dr. Cadieux is a practicing geriatric psychiatrist in Hershey, Pennsylvania. He serves as an editor, writer, and reviewer of geriatric and psychiatric publications.

Trademarks

Part 1

Seeing Aging Through Your Parents' Eyes

Not until you walk in someone else's shoes do you really understand what that person is going through or how he or she sees the world. As a baby boomer, you're closing in on what it feels like to be aging, but that's no substitute for being your parent's age.

In this part we give you a glimpse of what your parents see: how much their bodies are changing, the ageist prejudice they encounter, and what it's like to live in fear of cancer, heart attacks, brain attacks (strokes), and Alzheimer's. Even though some of these fears may be unfounded, it's important for you to know the symptoms and the actual likelihood that your mom and dad could encounter one of the many age-related conditions we review.

Chapter 1

Aging as Your Parent Sees It

In This Chapter

- Living in a society that worships youth
- Shifting family roles
- Seniors and independence
- Underlying fears of aging
- The upside to growing older
- The "sandwich generation"

Not until I survived the terrible twos with my kids did I really begin to appreciate my parents. Pretty amazing how parents get smarter, the older we get.

But few of us can grasp what it must be like to be *old:* To come to terms with aging, the change of roles, and the changes in a body you thought you knew. Before you begin caring for your mom and dad, step back a moment and get in touch with what they must be going through.

Living in an Ageist Society

When was the last time you stood at the grocery check out and saw countless pictures of healthy, hip older women and men on the front cover of trendy magazines? (Sorry, Paul Newman doesn't count.) We live in a culture that worships youth. Clothing, cosmetics, and lifestyle manufacturers trip over themselves trying to reach the youth market. Even when cosmetics are targeted to older women, they're hyped as "anti-aging" products. Popular television shows depict older people as senile, cranky, quirky, and suffering from a long list of ailments.

If you're a woman, it's considered cute to lie about your age. In fact, it's in poor taste to ask a woman her age, suggesting she should be ashamed of the answer. And there's nothing like black candles to make someone turning 50 realize he or she should be in mourning. Plastic surgery and hair transplants rescue those who find the *aging look* unbecoming.

The results of ageism go much deeper. Countless studies have shown how elderly patients are frequently misdiagnosed because their complaints are considered "normal." Depression, for example, goes unchecked despite the fact that suicide rates among older men rank highest in the nation. (I'll tell you more about that in Chapter 4, "Not-So-Normal Aging: The Mental Side.") Despite the fact that the Age Discrimination in Employment Act (ADEA) prohibits age discrimination in the workplace, older workers are often passed over for promotions, cutting short a fulfilling career. New training programs aren't even offered to older workers under the premise that "you can't teach an old dog new tricks." (Yet seniors are the fastest-growing group on the Internet!) Nearly 20,000 lawsuits are filed each year claiming age discrimination.

Geri-Fact

There are three age segments among the older population: young-old: 65 to 74 years; middle-old: 75 to 84 years; and old-old: 85+ years. People in each group grew up with different life experiences that shaped their world view. You won't find them thinking alike.

Besides being assaulted by a youth culture, your parents face a number of life changes that dramatically affect their view of life:

- Retirement from a long-held job may mean a loss of status, income, and the network of relationships held at work.

- As their children become adults with families of their own, Mom and Dad experience much less daily contact and interaction with their children.

- Spouses, friends, and siblings die, leaving older people to grieve over the loss of significant relationships.

- Chronic illnesses and changes in physical appearance cause your parents to see themselves differently, literally.

All of these changes can rock anyone's self-confidence. So when you initiate a caregiving role with your parent, do it ever so gently.

Change of Roles

My guess is that if you bought this book, your parents need you to take a more active role in their lives. Perhaps, it's to help them find the right physician, track down community services, or figure out what kind of housing options make sense for them. Maybe you're considering having your mom come to live with you or it's time to find a good nursing home for your dad.

Parent-child relationships are pretty complex (as if you didn't know). Some small remark from your dad can reduce you to a two year old. You may feel that your parents have somehow escaped the fact that you're now a 50-year-old woman with a career and grown kids. Instead, you're stuck in the middle-child slot or you're still the "baby" in the family. You may need to invite them into your adult world. It may seem like you're regressing with "show and tell" but show them examples of your work, or take them to your place of work. Today, there are so many different kinds of careers that your parents may truly not understand what you do. As a result, their images of you may be frozen in time.

Senior Alert

You are never your parent's parent. Your role as the adult child may change and evolve, but it doesn't mean that you and your parents switch roles and they become the child, no matter how dependent or mind-impaired they become. Treating your parent as your child undercuts their self-esteem and erodes the respect due your parent.

As your mom or dad becomes more dependent, the roles of all family members will shift. The youngest child who has expertise in an area where your parent needs help (for example, one of you is an insurance agent or a nurse) might become the leader of the group—a position that the eldest child might have held for years. The sibling who is in a position to take Mom to all of her doctor's appointments may be the one to organize the rest of the family around Mom's medical care. The son who has taken Dad in to live with him may be given more of an authoritative role among other family members in making future decisions *with* Dad and on his behalf. All of you need to be prepared for this shift. Trying to hold on to things "just like they've always been" will cause a great deal of frustration and denial. Families, just like any other group, thrive on balance. You've reached a comfort-zone in knowing everyone's place and in maintaining patterns of behavior you've grown accustomed to over the years. But your parent's *place* will change as he or she becomes more dependent. And similar to musical chairs, so will the *places* of the rest of the family members.

How you accept and appreciate your parents' aging is a critical piece to any caregiving role you assume. It will set the tone and direction of your evolving relationship with your parents. The more you understand the nature of any disease they are coping with or the life stages they are going through, the better off you'll be in knowing how to react. If Dad is accusing you of stealing from him and he is in the second stage of Alzheimer's, you'll feel better knowing that this is a common occurrence among those afflicted with the disease. It may still hurt you, but it takes the personal sting out of the accusation. Rather than react in a fit of anger against your dad, you can learn a more appropriate response. The goal of this book is to better prepare you for the vast array of caregiving opportunities and situations that you're going to find yourself in.

Fight for Independence

So you thought you were done with balancing acts: career and family, school and work. Get ready for a new act: balancing your parents' need for independence against their safety. How long should your dad drive? What do you do when you know it's not safe for him to be behind the wheel and he's adamant about driving? What do you do when Mom leaves the gas stove on, and gets lost in the neighborhood? Do you patch a network of services together so she can stay at home? Or should she move to an assisted living facility? As Mom recovers from hip surgery, when do you encourage her to start walking and when is she ready to get back to living on her own? (Part 3, "Understanding You and Your Parent's Options," can help you find answers to these questions.)

We live in a culture that respects independence. Most older people report that they don't want to be a burden to their families. Though they appreciate their children's offers to help, most parents want to retain their power and caretaking positions they've long held in the family. Chapter 11, "Remaining at Home: Making It Work," identifies a range of strategies that can safely help your parents remain independent. It will be important to support their need for independence and foster it to keep them active and well.

Geri-Fact

One of the most popular reasons older people give for buying long-term care insurance is "I don't want to be a burden to my kids. I don't want to depend on anybody."

As competent adults, Mom and Dad have the right to take risks and even make mistakes. Just as they had to let go when you were a teenager, you'll need to do the same for them. Of course, if they cross over into territory where they pose a safety hazard for themselves or others, you'll need to intervene.

Fears

The line "I've fallen and I can't get up" from a popular television commercial has become the brunt of many a joke. But the company using the ad was pretty smart. They knew that one of the greatest fears of the elderly is falling. Older people worry that they'll fall on ice, fall down steps, trip on broken sidewalks, or fall in the bathroom.

To make this fear even worse, they fear that no one will know they've fallen at home if they live alone. It's not unusual for older folks to restrict their physical activity because of this fear. The problem is, this strategy causes them to become isolated, lonely, and out of shape—all of which will make them more frail and more likely to do the one thing they fear—fall.

Because Mom might feel frail and vulnerable, she may find herself more fearful than she ever has in the past: She sees teenagers walking toward her in the mall as a gang about to steal her purse; Dad stops answering the door because he's afraid someone will rob him.

Senior Alert

Fears of falling aren't unfounded. According to the American Academy of Orthopaedic Surgeons, nearly one third of people over the age of 65 fall each year. Ninety percent of the 300,000 hip fractures treated annually in the U.S. occur as a result of a fall. This year alone there will be an estimated 350,000 fractures—nearly 1,000 hip fractures a day. Osteoporosis, especially among women, is a major culprit in falls. But so are hazards in the home such as poor lighting, sliding throw rugs, cluttered hallways, and slippery bathroom floors. Medications that make people dizzy or cause them to get up in the middle of the night to go to the bathroom are also culprits.

Besides worrying about falls and threats from the outside world, your parents worry about their bodies as they watch friends get diagnosed with cancer or Alzheimer's or suffer a stroke (which we'll cover in Chapters 5, "Brain Attacks (Strokes) and Heart Attacks," and 6, "Alzheimer's Disease and Cancer"). They live in fear that this could happen to them or their spouse. A constant dose of television doesn't help matters either: Watching daytime talk shows in which so many American families appear to be dysfunctional or listening to a constant stream of unsettling news lead many elderly viewers to think that the world has become a dangerous and unfamiliar place. Many retreat and withdraw. If they live alone and don't have a chance to interact with a healthy, functional outside world, their fears become all the more real, especially when they feel so vulnerable physically. That's why it's so important for your parents to remain active by joining friends in social events, getting out to a senior center, finding a part-time job, or volunteering. By staying engaged, they'll maintain balance in their lives. For ideas on how your mom and dad can remain

Senior Alert

Don't underestimate the power of fear: Older people die every year from heat waves in inner cities because they'd rather keep their windows shut from fear of having someone break in. Others fear a high electric bill and keep the air conditioning shut off.

active and independent, see Chapter 12, "Living in the Community: Services and Transportation."

Be aware of your parent's underlying fears, which may embarrass them and cause them to withdraw from an active lifestyle. You might be thinking Mom and Dad are just going through a phase or are no longer interested. My dad stopped going out to eat, which he loved doing, because he had a digestive problem and was so afraid of needing to get to the bathroom. It took us awhile to figure out what was going on. Once his digestive disorder was corrected with medication and diet changes, he was back on the restaurant scene enjoying himself and acting a lot less depressed.

The Upside of Aging

By now you're thinking, what's up with the *golden years*? Aging sure seems like quite a downer. But to the contrary, there are many positive aspects in growing older. For those who make the transition, they reach a stage of peace and contentment. They are at peace with who they are and what they've done with their lives. Erik Erikson, a famous psychoanalyst who has studied life stages, explains that one of the characteristics of a well-adjusted older person is what he calls "generativity"—a deep concern about the welfare of the next generation. Individuals who reach this phase are able to move beyond their own needs. They no longer are consumed with careers, the demands of "making it," and being absorbed with themselves (pretty nice place to be). There's plenty of evidence that lots of folks have reached this plateau—most of the millions of volunteers throughout this country are the elderly.

Most people love being a grandparent, they enjoy their leisure time, and many discover new hobbies that tap their creative juices. Be sure to encourage your parents to continue exploring and staying in good physical shape. Play to the upside in aging.

You're Not Alone

There's a myth out there that most of the elderly in this country live in nursing homes. The truth is, it's only a fraction of the population—4 percent at any given time. The majority live at home, in the community, or with relatives. The greatest amount of caregiving is given by family members and friends.

Women represent 75 percent of the caregivers, most of whom are spouses and daughters. According to the Administration on Aging (the federal government's agency on aging affairs), the average primary caregiver is female, 46 years old, married, works full-time, and is also caring for at least one child. It's no wonder she's been referred to as part of the "sandwich generation"—caught between caring for dependent children and dependent parents. Of course, not all caregivers fit this profile. Many are older women in their 60s and 70s caring for an ailing spouse. And here's a surprise: The oldest caregivers are husbands, nearly half being over the age of 75 years.

Silver Lining

Many companies are recognizing the value of older employees, especially in jobs that need part-time workers and that don't require heavy lifting. According to the Department of Labor, the number of people age 55 and over who remain in the workforce has jumped by six million since 1950. And to everyone's surprise, older people are catching on to information technology. Now, add to that skill a reliable work ethic from the Depression generation, and you have a terrific employee!

Overall, there are about 22 million caregivers of aging family members throughout the nation today. And those numbers aren't dwindling anytime soon. Breakthroughs in cancer research, Alzheimer's, and other age-related diseases, along with advances in genome research, will push the envelope on how long we live. Baby boomers who today find themselves in caregiving roles, are already beginning to experience their own aging.

You'll learn throughout this book that there are a great number of resources available to you in caring for your parents. The field is changing every day with new resources and new challenges. My goal is to make caregiving easier for you by cutting through the clutter and connecting you to the tools and support you'll need.

The Least You Need to Know

- Living in a society that values youth, and experiencing life changes such as retirement, can affect your parents' view of life.

- As your parent becomes more dependent, the roles of all family members begin to shift; however, "parenting your parent" is never healthy.

- It's important to balance your parents' need for independence against their safety.

- Chronic illnesses, fear of injury, less involvement in their children's lives, retirement, living in a youth culture, and the death of spouses, siblings, and friends are challenges aging parents face.

- Many older people reach a place of peace and contentment with their lives, giving back to younger generations. Don't let your parents miss this opportunity.

- The majority of seniors live at home, in the community, or with relatives, not in nursing homes. The greatest amount of caregiving is given by family members and friends.

Getting to Know a Different Body

Remember when you first had kids? How you'd read everything you could get your hands on to know just where your child fell on the developmental charts? Sure, you acted like it really didn't matter. But admit it. You loved knowing how your child was crawling ahead of schedule, talking up a storm before most other kids, and of course, took to potty training before *Sesame Street*'s Count Dracula could count to three. (Okay, maybe to 10.)

Wanting to be normal and, whenever possible, being better than normal is a lifetime pursuit. Until we hit aging. Then, all of a sudden, our ideas of what's normal and what's not are turned upside down. If it's *normal* to get Alzheimer's, have multiple bypass surgery, and have your hip replaced, then forget it. Who needs to be normal?

The Aging Explosion

The truth is most of us don't know what normal aging really looks like. There hasn't been a Dr. Spock out there giving us mileposts along the way. But Dr. Spock had millions of little kids to study. Everybody was doing it—going through childhood, that is. But how do you find millions of people living to 100 years old or even 80? They just haven't been around. But today, thanks to things like healthier lifestyles and medical breakthroughs, people are living longer than ever before. Humankind has never seen anything quite like it. Check out these numbers:

- In 1950 there were 200 million people in the world 60 years and older. That number has almost tripled today at 590 million, and in the next 25 years the number will top 1 billion. The whole world is going gray!

- By the year 2004 there will be an estimated 140,000 centenarians in the United States—the folks who've made it to 100 years old.

- The average American lives to 76 years old; in the 1920s you were making the news if you lived to 60.

Geri-Fact

When President Franklin D. Roosevelt gave us Social Security back in 1935, his budget gurus set the "normal" retirement age at 65 years because (you got it) few people reached that age in the first place. They knew how not to break the bank.

With our parents enjoying a normal life span of 76 years, and baby boomers (those of us born between 1946 and 1960) expecting to surpass that, we've got a bit of a budget problem with Social Security when our kids retire. But that's a topic for another book. Let's get back to figuring out just what is *normal* aging.

Two Kinds of Aging

The folks who have been studying aging have identified two kinds of aging: primary and secondary. Your parents don't get to pick which one. They're going to experience both.

Primary Aging

Primary aging is genetic. It's that part of aging where your parents are essentially along for the ride. It's the preprogrammed coding that their bodies follow. Some people have great genes and live a long time with a full head of hair.

No matter how great their genes, your parents will experience a decline in something known as trophic factors. Basically, these are the hormonal substances our bodies produce like estrogen, testosterone, and human growth factors. When Mom or Dad's body starts producing *less* of these, you start to see the classic signs of aging: less smooth skin, less hair, less hair color, and even less height. There's less bone mass and lost muscle fiber. And Mom or Dad's senses also become less effective. Hearing, vision, touch, smell, and even taste begin to decline, continuing on a downward descent as your parents age. Perhaps, one of the most damaging factors in primary aging is the immune system's inability to keep pace with past performance levels. It, too, becomes less effective leaving Mom and Dad susceptible to the flu, pneumonia, and any other infections that come along.

Secondary Aging

Here's where your parents get to take some control over their aging. A lifestyle of moderate exercise, no smoking, a healthy diet, and staying active can delay the effects of secondary aging caused by the systems of the body simply slowing down. The circulatory system becomes less efficient and the heart gets sluggish. The vessels that carry the blood to and from the heart become clogged and constricted. Lungs lose nearly half of their capacity by the time your parent turns 80 and the muscular-skeletal system loses its strength, giving way to stiff joints and weak muscles. This slowing down of the body's systems also affects digestion because it takes longer for food to pass through Dad's system. He will also absorb food and fluids at an erratic rate, which for most people is slower. Overall, Dad's body will work just fine at this slower pace. Pushing his body beyond its capacity, however, will get him in trouble.

Since we're on this "slow but sure" theme, let's not leave out the brain. The *speed* of processing information by the brain is diminished with age; however, the *quality* of thinking—the ability to learn and remain intelligent—does *not* naturally decrease with age.

Silver Lining

Research studies show that our ability to understand, reflect, and interpret information actually *increases* with age. That's why cultures throughout history have revered their elders for their wisdom—a word we seldom associate with the young. In fact, the U.S. Senate derives its name from the Latin word *senatus,* meaning "elder," the assumption being that to qualify for the senate, you need the kind of judgment that only old age brings.

Aging: Everybody's Doing It

So what changes can any normal person over 60 expect from his or her body? There are quite a few changes, and of course, everybody's different, but in the rest of this chapter I'll tell you about the five most common changes.

The Vision Thing

Notice how fashionable those drug store reading glasses are becoming? They're even sold at the trendy bookstores where you might have picked up this book. It might have something to do with the fact that millions of baby boomers are experiencing one of the first signs of aging.

As we age, the lens of the eye begins to become more rigid, which leads to a form of farsightedness called presbyopia, in which the eye cannot focus easily on close objects. By the time your parents are in their 60s and 70s this condition becomes much more pronounced. They will also be noticing other changes. Glare, especially from headlights can actually blind them and certainly pose problems for nighttime driving. They'll find it difficult to see in dimly lit rooms and hallways. Refocusing takes longer when they're going from light to dark rooms. It's harder to distinguish between colors. Contrasts and shadows become more difficult to decipher making it troublesome to go down steps or walk along sidewalks.

Most of these vision problems can be dealt with by making sure the halls are well lit in your parents' home, that the house isn't a cluttered obstacle course, especially in high traffic areas, and that your parents get annual eye exams. As read about in Chapter 3, "Not-So-Normal Aging: The Physical Side," older people can develop some very serious vision problems. Their eyesight is far too precious for them to lose.

What Did You Say?

My kids and husband are getting pretty tired of me saying, "What?" I complain that they're all mumbling or there's too much noise in the background. But I know the real reason—it's just hard to admit it when I've just turned 50. But hey, there's President Clinton sporting a hearing aid. Of course, he has a cool reason for it: too many loud concerts in the 1960s.

The fact of the matter is, hearing loss begins earlier than we think. By the time your parents and their friends made it to their 60s—one out of three

Geri-Fact

As we age, nerve and sensory cells of the inner ear decline and die off. As a result, auditory signals to the brain aren't relayed. The damage to the ear doesn't really affect your parent's ability to pick up the volume of sounds. What it does affect is the ability to *distinguish* sounds. Consonants such as "s," "f," and "p" are hard to pick up, and so are high-pitched sounds.

already had significant hearing loss. Half of everyone over 75 years has a real hard time hearing. Men are affected more than women. Lot's of researchers think that being exposed to loud sounds throughout life has a lot to do with hearing loss. It's that slow, bit-by-bit nature of losing his hearing that lulls Dad into thinking he really hasn't lost it yet. Certainly not enough to make him want to buy a hearing aid.

Nerve deafness will cause your parent to confuse words that sound alike. A conversation like this might take place:

> You: "Hey Mom, it's time to take your pill."

> Mom: "Fill? Okay dear, I'll fill your coffee in a minute."

Background noise blurs hearing even more. So talking in a restaurant, at a family gathering, or with a TV in the background makes it doubly hard for older people to understand what you and their friends are saying.

When carrying on a conversation becomes real work, you'll find Dad starting to withdraw rather than deal with the hassle. You also might find him getting argumentative because he misunderstands what you're saying. And you'll find yourself withdrawing, too. You'll start yelling at him because you think that pumping up the volume is the answer. But it's not a volume problem, so he takes your talking louder as an insult. He just can't figure out what you're saying. You both end up annoyed. Besides, the more you raise your voice, the higher pitched your voice becomes, making it harder for him to distinguish sounds.

Even though everybody suffers hearing loss associated with age, getting Dad to get his hearing checked may hit a wall of resistance. A hearing aid is like a neon sign flashing **OLD MAN.** It's an old stigma that really needs to go. Focus on what he's losing out on. The conversations with his grand kids, the fact that the two of you are talking less to each other, and how Mom is missing their old dinner conversations. Let him know that hearing aids aren't what they used to be when *his* Dad used one. They're a lot smaller and well hidden. Some of the new hearing aids (I have one) are computerized and automatically adjust the background noise. The audiologist can specifically lower sounds that you personally find annoying, such as the clattering of dishes in a restaurant (or my teenagers asking for my ATM card). The new technology is amazing. Don't let your parents make a decision not to get a hearing aid based on outdated stereotypes!

An exam by a physician might reveal that your Dad doesn't need a hearing aid, after all. (Another reason to convince him to go to the doctor.) Older folks build up thicker and drier earwax. Too much of this in front of Dad's eardrum will cause hearing loss, so he might just need a good old ear cleaning. Or he might have excess fluid in the inner ear, an ear infection, or a hereditary condition. Some of these conditions can be corrected through surgery or medication. Only a specialized physician can determine the best course for your parent.

Senior Alert

Make sure Mom and Dad have their hearing checked by a physician who is a specialist in hearing. An otolaryngologist or otologist can determine any physical reasons causing your parents' hearing loss. The physician might then refer Mom or Dad to a certified audiologist who has graduate training in hearing impairment and will be able to determine the degree of hearing loss your parent is experiencing. Don't assume it's an "age thing" and take your parent to people who sell hearing aids as your first step.

If Dad does get a hearing aid, don't expect him to take to it like a fish to water. It takes getting used to and some training. One in four people who try out hearing aids, end up stashing them in their bedroom dresser. So make sure Dad sees someone who will give him training and offers at least a 30-day trial. Plan on taking him back at least once to fine-tune the device. And by the way, Medicare does *not* cover hearing aids. Shop around for price.

Here are some tips to help you make hearing easier for your parents:

- Talk a little slower, not louder.
- Take the time to pronounce your words.

Sage Source

Self Help for Hard of Hearing People is a nonprofit, educational organization that offers good links and information and identifies free screening sites throughout the country during annual Hearing Loss Week. Contact them at 7910 Woodmont Avenue, Suite 1200, Bethesda, MD 20814; 301-657-2248; www.shhh.org.

- Hold the same level of conversation you've always had; in other words, don't talk down to them.
- Start the conversation with the subject you're going to talk about: "Hey, Dad, about that ballgame last night." When you change the subject, introduce the new topic, "And another thing Dad, let's talk about Mom's birthday."
- Use facial expressions and gestures: Point, touch, nod.
- Make sure you are both looking at each other.
- Cut down background noise: Shut off the TV, radio, or dishwasher, and at restaurants search for the quieter spots.
- Don't ramble. Use direct, straightforward sentences and pause a moment between them.

- Make sure there's enough light so you can see each other and that it's not shining in their eyes.

I've Had It with Counting Sheep!

I can still hear my mom telling me to come in from a great game of hide 'n' seek because it was bedtime. "But Mom, ..." and she'd retort with, "You need your eight hours of sleep." Now, I'm here years later with a teenage son who needs 10 hours (I just wish it wasn't *during* school). Growing bodies do need a good amount of sleep to recharge those Energizer Bunny bodies of theirs. But the older body sleeps less soundly. On average it will take Dad longer to fall asleep and he'll sleep lighter than he did in his younger days. He might nap more, but it's light sleep that he's getting.

One reason for this drop in restful, restorative sleep is that there are fewer brain cells in charge of deep sleep. There are five stages of sleep, with the deep, restorative stages being the third and fourth stage. Older people seem to get less of this. They also tend to experience less R.E.M. (rapid eye movement) sleep, which is the fifth stage—the kind that has your eyes flickering while you're dreaming. All that flickering causes an increased blood supply and the flow of some mighty fine brain chemicals. You can thank these guys for that restored, *I'm out to conquer the world* feeling when you wake up. (Really, Starbucks doesn't deserve the credit.)

When the body ages, there's less melatonin, the hormone that's been found to regulate sleep. If Mom is in her 70s or 80s the levels may be barely traceable. Besides these physical changes, getting little exercise, drinking caffeine, and smoking all contribute their fair share in robbing your parents of a good night's sleep.

Your parents might not be too happy with their new sleep patterns. If they stubbornly stay in bed until they get a full night's sleep they'll never win. The key is to find ways to make sleep more effective and wake up feeling refreshed. Mom or Dad might have to invest more time and care in making this happen.

Here are some tips to help your parents get a good night's sleep:

- Develop a regular, soothing routine for going to bed, such as listening to music, reading, or visualizing a favorite place like the beach. This is a great time for a massage, a warm bath, or putting on skin lotion.

Geri-Fact

It's a myth that older people need *less* sleep. Adult sleep needs, according to the National Sleep Foundation, remain constant throughout most of our lives. Most of us will require seven to nine hours of sleep throughout our lifetime. It's the stages of sleep that will undergo change.

- Stick to the same bedtime and naptime every day. A consistent schedule helps set Mom and Dad's biological clocks and cues their bodies that it's time to sleep.

- Exercise in the early afternoon, not right before bedtime.

- Drink hardly any fluids a few hours before bedtime so there's no need to go to the bathroom in the middle of the night.

- Stay clear of coffee, tea, cola, and other caffeine-laden drinks or foods eight hours before bedtime.

- Keep daytime napping limited to afternoons, not late in the day, and no longer than an hour. Watch out for dozing off in front of the TV.

- Avoid heavy meals close to bedtime especially those that are spicy. Dinners around 5:00 P.M. give adequate time for digestion.

- Ask the doctor about the side effects of certain prescription drugs, which can cause sleeping problems. Perhaps the dosage or time of day to take the drug can be changed.

- Don't smoke. Besides a zillion other reasons not to smoke, nicotine plays havoc with sleep.

- Avoid alcohol at bedtime. Although it may appear to put you to sleep, Mom or Dad will actually awaken early without feeling restored.

Even though there are normal changes with sleep patterns as Mom and Dad age, don't dismiss your Dad's complaints of not getting enough sleep. If he isn't feeling rested when he gets up in the morning there may be other problems, such as coronary artery disease, lung disease, thyroid problems, depression, anxiety, or dementia. Side effects of medications are another culprit. Don't brush off sleeping problems as just "part of the package" with old age. Your dad should describe his sleeping problems to his physician, who will then explore all of the possibilities behind Dad's sleeping problems. Don't let him simply walk out of the doctor's office with sleeping pills in hand thinking the problem is solved.

Sage Source

A great way of keeping track of sleep patterns that your parent can share with their doctor is to get a copy of the National Sleep Foundation's sleep diary. Call 202-347-3471 or visit their Web site at www.sleepfoundation.org.

Let's talk about sleeping pills for a moment. When I was Secretary of Aging for the state of Pennsylvania, I was responsible for a prescription program for about 400,000 elderly. After a national television show exposed the side effects of the drug Halcion, a popular sleeping pill, we did some research of our own. We discovered that thousands of our cardholders had been taking sleeping pills for *years*. Now, any good doctor will tell you that sleeping pills are meant to be taken for only a very short period of time—we're talking days, *maybe* a week or two. Even the drug companies that manufacture the pills recommend temporary usage. Yet despite all the cautions against it, 40 percent of all patients in this country who are taking hypnotic drugs to sleep are over 65 years. Yet, your parents' age group makes up only 12 percent of the population. Yikes. Plenty of research has backed up the National Institute of Aging's claim that "hypnotic medication should *not* be the *mainstay* of management for most of the causes of disturbed sleep."

Senior Alert

Taking sleeping pills for the long haul can cause daytime sleepiness, anxiety, cognitive (thinking) decline, and falls. Getting off the drug must be done very carefully. If this is the case for your parent, work with a physician to gradually and safely oversee your parent's withdrawal of the drug.

The Hot and Cold of It

The brain's thermostat starts to lose its sensitivity to picking up temperature changes as we age. Folks in their mid-80s find this especially troublesome. Complicating this are circulatory problems and medications that can throw your parents' thermostats out of whack. You also lose your ability to sweat in old age, so now your parents are left without nature's protective cooling system.

Your parents probably grew up without air conditioning and it was a badge of honor to be able to "take the heat." So there's your mom out in the garden in 80 degree heat and your dad pushing the lawn mower. Not a good scenario. During my stint as Secretary of Aging, we were hit with a heat wave in Philadelphia and more than 100 people more than 60 years of age died of heat-related deaths due to *hyperthermia*. Many were found in their homes with their windows shut because they were afraid of people breaking in, or they kept the AC off to avoid high utility bills. We learned from that experience and launched a prevention program with senior centers and the Area Agency on Aging. It's made a great difference in Philly, but every year with more heat waves throughout the country, thousands of elderly people are overcome with heat stroke. During a heat wave, be sure to check on your parents.

Geri-Fact

Hyperthermia means a body temperature that is dangerously high, while **hypothermia** means a body temperature that is dangerously low.

Here are some tips for helping your parents cope with the heat:

- Make sure they're drinking plenty of fluids.
- Make sure they keep the air conditioning on, but older people should not be sitting right in front of it—their bodies could cool off too much and then they'll suffer *hypothermia.*
- If they're using a fan, make sure a window is open to create a draft rather than simply circulating hot air in a closed room like an oven.
- If they don't have air conditioning, suggest they spend the day at the mall. Or how about buying your parents an air conditioner *and* arranging to pay for the extra electricity?
- Suggest they take a lukewarm bath or shower; it's one of the best ways to cool off.
- Call or visit twice a day—if Mom or Dad starts acting confused, has a headache, is dizzy, or is nauseous, your parent is showing signs of a heat stroke. Call for medical help.
- Suggest Mom or Dad keep a cool cloth around the back of the neck.

On the other hand, your mom and dad are also vulnerable to becoming too cold and can lapse into hypothermia. Of course, this is a more likely problem in the winter but they can also become victims by sitting in front of an air conditioner. Room temperatures lower than 65 degrees can induce hypothermia. During cool nights make sure your parents have warm bedclothes and blankets because they are more likely to lose body heat while they're sleeping.

Both hyperthermia and hypothermia are medical emergencies. The weather can pose a real danger to your parents—watch out for them.

Now, Why Did I Go to the Store?

Billions of the brain's nerve cells bite the dust between adolescence and old age. The brain also becomes smaller and lighter. By the time Mom has reached 90, as much as half of her original nerve cells are lost. It sounds pretty dismal, but it's not. I like to think of it as clearing out some space on my hard drive. Who needs 85 years of files, anyway?

What's normal is that she might be more forgetful than she ever was and she may be a bit slower. But in no way does that mean she has lost her intelligence. When you look up a number in the phone book, close it, and then dial, you're using short-term memory. Without much fanfare, you decided that you weren't going to store it in your head. It's that kind of memory—the kind that you have in mind for the short term—that older folks have more difficulty retaining. And if they want to store this new information into long-term memory, they have to work a little harder than the rest of us to retrieve it. Retrieving stored data is going to take more time. Your parents shouldn't panic if they experience short-term forgetfulness or if they aren't slamming the buzzer as fast as they used to playing along with *Jeopardy*.

Even though you might find Mom or Dad calculating a waiter's tip slower than he or she did before, or not making a quick decision when there are multiple choices, don't go off making the same mistake you did as a teenager—they really are pretty smart people. And they can get smarter. Just like your aerobics instructor yells out, "Use it or lose it," keeping mentally active can help Mom and Dad stay mentally fit—as in, "He might be old but his mind is as sharp as a tack." Hey, one of the fastest-growing groups on the Internet is more than 60!

However, if you suspect that your parent is actually confused and forgetting very common, important facts in his or her life, you'll find help in Chapter 6, "Alzheimer's Disease and Cancer."

The Least You Need to Know

- We experience both primary aging (changes caused by genetics) and secondary aging (caused by the systems of the body slowing down). We can control some of the aging process by choosing a healthy lifestyle.

- Presbyopia (difficulty in seeing things close to you) is the most common vision problem due to aging.

- Before your parent buys a hearing aid, make sure he or she sees a physician first to determine what's causing the loss.

- Sleeping patterns change with age. Your parents need as much sleep as they always did, but they'll be getting less deep sleep.

- Hyperthermia and hypothermia can be life threatening; the elderly are especially vulnerable.

- The older mind takes a bit longer to process and retrieve information, but that doesn't mean older folks have any less intelligence.

Chapter 3

Not-So-Normal Aging: The Physical Side

In This Chapter

- Dealing with incontinence
- How your mom and dad's vision is at risk as they age
- Diabetes: not just for kids
- Osteoporosis and arthritis
- Smoking and chronic obstructive pulmonary disease (COPD)

There are some common health problems that your parents and their friends find all too familiar. That doesn't mean these conditions are normal—they're just common. When you were raising your kids, it wasn't uncommon to hear about a child having tonsillitis or having so many earaches that the child needed to have tubes put in. However, these problems aren't normal.

Same deal with your parents. There are some common ailments and conditions that many older people face. But that doesn't make them normal. So when your mom hints to you about being incontinent, or has become extremely withdrawn, don't make the mistake of quietly thinking to yourself, "She's 80, what else can you expect?" But many of these conditions are not par for the course. And with proper intervention, these conditions can be improved, made easier to live with, and in some case can be completely reversed.

Hard to Hold: Incontinence

When June Lockhart of *Lassie* fame starred in an adult briefs commercial, *urinary incontinence* officially came out of the closet. Even though it's refreshing to see this condition out in the open, it has also portrayed incontinence as normal for old age. It gives the impression that you simply treat this yourself by grabbing for the adult briefs at the grocery store or have them discretely sent to you through the mail. It also makes people think that there's really nothing that can be done about it. They are wrong on both counts.

Incontinence, though it affects at least 13 million Americans, is not normal. It's definitely a sisterhood thing: 85 percent of people affected by incontinence are women. Before Mom resigns herself to adult briefs she needs to be seen by her family doctor or urologist to determine the cause of the disorder. Medications, an acute illness, a urinary tract infection or endocrine problems can all cause incontinence. It could also be the symptom of an underlying disease, and that's why she needs a physician to do the detective work to find out what's really going on. There also might be a weakening of the muscles supporting the urinary tract.

Geri-Fact

Urinary incontinence is the uncontrollable loss of urine. It can occur at any age, with the causes tending to be different for each age group. The likelihood of urinary incontinence increases with age. About one out of every three seniors over 60 have some type of bladder control problem.

There are three major types of incontinence:

- **Stress incontinence.** The muscles of the pelvic floor, which have been dutifully supporting the bladder for all these years, become weakened—mostly due to the wear and tear of childbirth and menopause's hormonal changes. The bladder slips down without the muscle support and now the abdominal muscles can squeeze the bladder. So whenever Mom coughs, lifts something, strains, or sneezes, those abs put enough stress on the bladder to leak out urine.

- **Overflow incontinence.** Urine in the bladder builds up to a point where the muscle that controls the flow (urinary sphincter) can't hold it. Urine leaks out throughout the day. Men who have enlarged prostrates are especially vulnerable because the prostrate blocks the normal flow of urine causing it to hold up in the bladder until it overflows. Usually, there's no bladder sensation involved.

- **Urge incontinence.** Your parent will feel an urgent need to urinate and just not be able to hold it. There's hardly any time between feeling the need to void and actually urinating. This may be caused by an infection or medications. In this case, it can be reversed. But if Mom has had a stroke or suffers from dementia or another neurologic disorder, it can mean that the brain is no longer able to send the "hold off" signals to the bladder.

Chances are Mom won't be inclined to tell you about her incontinence. It's still a taboo topic for many people. Even physicians! Studies have found that many docs don't ask their older patients during exams about possible incontinence. And far too many doctors haven't had any training on how to treat it. So you really have to push on this one. Just letting your parents know how lots of their friends are probably going through the same thing, that it can be reversible, and that it could be a sign of something they don't want to ignore can help them get past the embarrassment factor.

Incontinence can be very isolating. Your mom or dad might stop going on trips, the movies, and outings with you or their friends because one of them lives in constant fear of having an accident. If you see a real drop in your parents' social activity, incontinence could be the reason. Gently explore it as a possibility.

What Can Be Done?

Incontinence can go away on its own but if it doesn't a doctor is the best one to determine the cause and course of action that's best. The treatment will vary according to what's wrong.

There are a number of steps your mom and dad can take on their own to cope with their incontinence:

- Get a schedule going. Schedule bathroom trips before experiencing the urge to urinate becomes too strong. Slowly extend the time between bathroom trips to train the bladder to "hold it."
- Make sure the pathway to the bathroom is clear. Getting there shouldn't be an obstacle course.
- If your parents have to negotiate steps to get to the bathroom, they should consider buying a portable commode, or if they can afford it, installing a second bathroom.
- Don't drink liquids three hours before going to bed.
- Eliminate drinks that irritate the bladder like caffeine in coffee, tea, and sodas. Alcoholic drinks also make this hit list.
- Stay clear of foods that are not bladder friendly like sugar, chocolate, spicy foods, and grapefruit.
- Take medications, especially diuretics, on a schedule that won't force Mom or Dad to get up in the middle of the night to urinate or wake up to soaked sheets. This can also save your parents from a nasty fall as they gropes to find their way to the toilet.
- When your parents are at an event, suggest to them that they find out where the restrooms are before they need them. Suggest they try to find seating closest to the restrooms.

- Mom can practice Kegel exercises, which means squeezing the muscles of the vagina and anus three times a day for 25 repetitions at five seconds each. To identify that muscle, Mom needs to try to stop the flow of urine in midstream. This exercise has proven to be very effective to help with mild cases of stress incontinence.

- Inhaling cigarette smoking irritates the bladder. Don't smoke and stay clear of secondhand smoke.

Sage Source

My best picks for help with incontinence are:

National Association for Continence
P.O. Box 8310
Spartanburg, SC 29305-8310
www.nafc.org

Simon Foundation for Continence
P.O. Box 815
Wilmette, IL 60091
1-800-23-SIMON

National Institute of Diabetes & Digestive & Kidney Diseases
31 Center Drive, MSC 2560
Bethesda, MD 20892-2560
www.niddk.nih.gov

Other Options

In the tougher cases of incontinence there are other options. Medications seem to help a great number of women. In general, these drugs help with urge incontinence that relax the bladder muscles to stop abnormal contractions. Some women, however, report that the side effects of these, such as anxiety medications, outweigh the benefit.

The FDA has reviewed and is expected to approve two new devices for stress incontinence in women. One device acts as a urethral plug about one fifth the size of a tampon and the other is a single-use foam pad a little bigger than a postage stamp. For some women this may be just the ticket, although they will have to watch for infections. The more serious intervention is surgery to remove a blockage, repair the urethra, or reposition the bladder. As a last resort catheters can be placed into the bladder through the urethra to drain the bladder. You'll need to be on the look out for infections with catheters, too.

If Mom decides that her best option is to wear adult briefs, she should be aware that she will be very vulnerable to skin infections and irritations. Learning how to keep her skin clean and dry is essential. Make sure there's an adequate supply in the house, so she won't hesitate to change them as frequently as she should.

Vision Under Attack

Four major eye diseases frequently afflict older people: cataracts, glaucoma, macular degeneration, and diabetic retinopathy. Here's what you should know about each.

Cataracts

If you want to get a sense of what it feels like to see with cataracts put some Vaseline on your reading glasses. Now try walking around. Most people with cataracts will tell you that they feel like they are looking through a cloud. That's because the transparent lens of the eye becomes filmy. All light that enters the eye passes through the lens. So if any part of the lens blocks, distorts, or diffuses the incoming light, then vision will be impaired. Cataracts can also block bright light from being diffused. The result? The trapped light touches off a fireworks display: halos around lights, scattering light, and glare. Not the kind of display you want in your eyeball!

Just about everybody over 65 years has cataracts—in most cases they are pretty mild and rarely painful. But when cataracts become severe and impair vision to a point where Mom or Dad can't perform daily tasks or feels unsafe, it's time to check out cataract surgery. The ophthalmologist will implant a new plastic or silicon lens. You'll need to make sure that your parent takes his or her eyedrops at the prescribed times and dutifully takes whatever other medication is prescribed. Today, the surgery is usually done at a day facility and Mom or Dad will leave with some pretty cool sunglasses.

Glaucoma

Glaucoma is sneaky. Your mom or dad probably won't complain of any problems until this culprit has done some pretty serious damage. We're talking partial or total blindness. The message? Parents need regular checkups just like your kids. Make sure they see a full-fledged physician (ophthalmologist) at least once a year.

Glaucoma is caused by pressure in the eyeball that increases to such a point that it damages the optic nerve. Once the damage is done you can't recover the lost vision. The pressure is caused by fluid inside the eyeball that fails to drain. This leads to a loss in peripheral vision—the ability to see things at your side. No one seems to know the actual cause of glaucoma but it does seem to run in families, especially among African-Americans and folks with diabetes. Treatment can range from medications to laser therapy and surgery. The goal is to stop the disease from getting worse.

Macular Degeneration

The macula is the central, most vital area of the retina. Its main job is to focus on fine details in the center of your field of vision. In other words, the macula goes on overload when you're searching for Waldo. When the macula starts degenerating, Mom might start complaining how straight lines are starting to appear wavy (see the Amsler Test in the following figure). She might also have blind spots that appear directly in front of what she's looking at. My mom has this condition, and she says it's like seeing around a small black hole.

If your mom or dad has this condition, you'll hear the terms wet or dry. If your parent has dry macular degeneration then a pigment is deposited in the macula with no scarring, blood, or other fluid leakage; if it's wet then there is leakage. Lots of times there are small hemorrhages surrounding the macula. In either case, both eyes are usually affected at the same time. Little treatment is available; however, when new blood vessels grow in or around the macula, laser surgery can sometimes destroy them from doing further harm. The good news is, this condition rarely causes total blindness. The bad news is, it can cause severe loss of vision.

Geri-Fact

If your parents have an optometrist—an eye and vision specialist who does not have a medical degree—make sure that person has a direct affiliation with a physician. The optometrist is trained to pick up major eye diseases, but treatment and diagnostic decisions should be made by an ophthalmologist.

This grid is known as the Amsler Test. If the line in the middle looks wavy to the person looking at it, that person might have macular degeneration and needs to see the eye doctor. An early diagnosis can stop further sight loss. It's a good idea to make a copy of this and tape it on your parents' bathroom mirror!

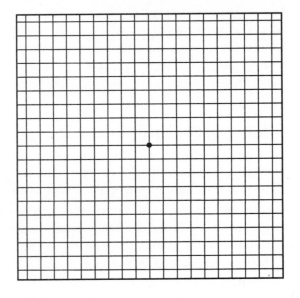

Diabetic Retinopathy

Diabetes plays havoc with the retina because high blood sugar levels make the walls of small blood vessels in the retina thicker, yet weaker, so they're more prone to deformity and leaks. This leads to blurred vision and if left untreated, blindness. The major lesson here is to keep those glucose levels controlled and blood pressure levels in the normal range. Again, an annual eye exam is mandatory for your parents if they're diabetic.

If your parents have any of these vision problems, find them a low vision specialist (usually an optometrist or ophthalmologist), who is trained in prescribing assistive devices to help people who are visually impaired.

Diabetes at Her Age?

We usually think of diabetes as a childhood disease. But nearly one in 12 people over 65 years come down with what is known as adult-onset, or Type 2, diabetes. Those of you with parents over 85 years should know that one in four will become diabetic. Now, if Mom and Dad are overweight and inactive, they're dramatically increasing their odds of becoming diabetic. Diabetes is the seventh highest cause of death among the elderly and the leading cause of blindness for those who are middle-aged and over. And it doesn't end there: with diabetes your mom's body (women get diabetes more often than men) can't regulate the level of glucose in her system. Without a regulator in charge, too little glucose reaches the body's cells. This badly affects their performance: They don't function or reproduce. On the other hand, too much glucose hangs out in the blood stream running amok throughout the body leaving in its wake: hardened arteries, damage to the retina, skin disorders, and a deteriorated nervous system.

Sage Source

The Lighthouse National Center for Vision and Aging (www.lighthouse.org) has helpful information for those with vision problems, and a terrific catalog of devices to make life easier and vision better. They can also tell you where a low vision clinic is located near you. Call 1-800-334-5497, or their TDD line, 212-808-5544. On their Web site you can see how your parent sees with glaucoma, diabetic retinopathy, and macular generation!

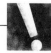

Senior Alert

The American Diabetes Association warns that just over half of the 11 million people who have adult-onset diabetes are even diagnosed with the disease and only one in four of those get proper treatment.

If Mom starts complaining of fatigue, weight loss, blurred vision, extreme hunger or thirst, and itchy skin, get her to a doctor. Not all older patients have the same classic symptom as kids—needing to urinate all of the time. So don't use this as your only barometer. Diabetes in older people creeps up on them with many of the symptoms being masked by the process of aging. Make sure your parents have a blood sugar level test (prick on the finger) as part of their annual cholesterol exams.

The doctor will probably recommend some lifestyle change—like losing weight, exercising, and following a diabetic diet. Insulin therapy might also be in order, which will stimulate insulin secretion to get those fuel levels regulated. Few patients take to this new routine like fish to water. Old habits, especially when they involve food, are hard to change. Become your mom's trainer and help with food preparation, exercising, and medications. If you're worried about Mom or Dad eating properly, hire someone (or do it yourself) to prepare meals for the week that are diabetic-friendly and freeze them in microwavable containers. Meals on Wheels programs also provide diabetic meals. Call your local senior center to find the program that's closest to your parents.

Be patient and monitor Mom's glucose. Today, there are self-monitoring kits with blood-testing meters. Also watch out for her foot care. Because she is vulnerable to nerve damage, she might not notice injuries on her feet. Infections can easily set in, placing her at risk for amputation.

Sage Source

An excellent Web site with links to plenty of other top-notch sites is by the National Institute of Diabetes & Digestive & Kidney Diseases at www.niddk.nih.gov. The American Diabetes Association is another great resource. Call them at 1-800-342-2383 or visit them on the Web at www.diabetes.org.

Osteoporosis

One in four women who are 65 years old will likely suffer a broken bone from *osteoporosis* by the time she reaches 85 years old. And one third of them will suffer a broken hip by age 90. Trust me, women aren't suffering these breaks because they're into extreme sports. It happens just getting out of bed, or even reaching for something. My mom has this condition and recently had a coughing spell leaving her with a broken rib. A slight fall on another occasion left her with a severely fractured wrist. Even though she fears a hip fracture, she stays active but has become much more cautious in her moving about.

Why are our mothers breaking their bones? Osteoporosis simply means porous bones. Ever buy coral for your goldfish bowl or aquarium? Mom's bones are pretty similar. They might seem hard but they are porous. The more porous the bone, the less dense it is, making the bone structurally weak. Like the coral, the bones feel hard but they are also brittle. All too often, we think of our bones like the skeletons clanging away at Halloween. But real-life skeletons are dynamic; they add and subtract calcium, rely on bone-building minerals, and are affected by hormones.

After menopause women lose bone mass. Most of the loss occurs the first 10 years after menopause. So, to any 50-year-olds reading this book who think that this is a 70s thing: You're wrong! From now on, calcium tablets should be on your shopping list. Taking calcium should become as second nature as brushing your teeth. The National Institutes of Health recommends that post-menopausal women should take 1,500 milligrams a day of calcium, along with vitamin D, which helps bones absorb calcium. Younger women should take 1,200 milligrams of calcium a day. Women who are at most risk are Caucasians (the fairer the complexion, the greater the risk), women who are thin and small-boned, those whose mothers had osteoporosis, and women who smoke, drink excessive alcohol, experience early menopause, or have taken prednisone (an anti-inflammatory steroidal drug).

Whatever your mom's age, she still can help her bones by taking calcium supplements, eating calcium rich foods, stopping smoking, and exercising. Lifting weights is great and so is walking, swimming, water aerobics, or riding a bike. Even at her age Mom can strengthen her bones. The two of you must also become watchdogs on preventing falls. Mom needs to stay home during ice storms (not everybody is a snowbird); get rid of throw rugs that take her on a magic carpet ride, landing her on her tail bone; wear nonskid shoes; ditch the floppy slippers; and make sure the steps are clear, well lit, and the hand rail is sturdy. For more on making the home a safer place, check out Chapter 11, "Remaining at Home: Making It Work."

Geri-Fact

Osteoporosis is a progressive decrease in the density of bones that weakens the bone. It is responsible for an annual 1.5 million fractures, including 300,000 hip fractures, 500,000 spinal fractures, and 200,000 wrist fractures. One third of all American women over 50 will have a spinal fracture. Osteoporosis is largely preventable with adequate calcium and exercise.

Sage Source

For more information, contact the National Osteoporosis Foundation, 1232 22nd Street NW, Washington, DC, 20037-1292; 202-223-2226; www.nof.org. Or contact the National Institutes of Health, Osteoporosis and Related Bone Diseases, 1232 22nd Street NW, Washington, DC 20037; 1-800-624-BONE; www.osteo.org.

Arthritis

Arthritis is a disease of the joints. *Arth* means "joint" and *itis* means "inflammation." Inflamed areas of the joints become red, swollen, stiff, and painful, causing a loss of mobility. The joints are made up of shock-absorbers known as cartilage positioned in between connecting bones. There seems to be two major reasons for this joint disease: The shock-absorbers wear thin from wear and tear just like the ones on your car, and joint tissues are broken down by biochemical changes in their composition.

Here are the basics on three of the most common arthritic conditions your mom or dad might face:

- **Osteoarthritis.** Cartilage in the joints has become extremely thin and frayed causing the joints to swell. Joints in the hands, feet, hips, knees, and back are it's usual victims. Every living being with a skeleton eventually comes down with this condition. But not everybody feels pain.

- **Rheumatoid arthritis.** This affects the whole body, not just a few joints. The immune system turns on the joints and attacks them. It also attacks other connective tissues in the tendons of the joints, heart, and lungs. It is a disease that will have dramatic flare ups making the joints extremely stiff and painful and then settle down. Symptoms start with flu-like symptoms of soreness, stiffness, achy joints, and fatigue. A specialist in managing this disease is highly recommended. Get your parent to a rheumatologist.

- **Gout.** More men are affected by this form of arthritis than women. It is extremely painful. The deal here is that uric acid, which didn't make its exit during urination, builds up and forms crystals in the joints. Your dad will get the message that these invaders are in his joints with sudden intense pain. The crystals head for the big toe, foot, ankle, knee, or wrist. The only good news here is that the assault comes and goes and lasts for a few days and then eventually fades over a week or two. People who get gout attacks need to watch the foods they eat, especially foods with a high purine content like beer and gravies. There are drugs (such as colchicine) that lessen the pain during an attack.

Sage Source

For more information, contact the Arthritis Foundation Information Line, 1-800-283-7800; www.arthritis.org. Or contact the American College of Rheumatology, 400-633-3777; www.rheumatology.org.

If your parents have any of these arthritic conditions, you're going to hear about NSAIDs (pronounced *N-sayds*). These are high-powered nonsteroidal anti-inflammatory drugs. Their job is to stop the production of prostaglandins, the culprit in causing Mom and Dad's joint swelling and pain.

NSAIDs can be extremely helpful but one side effect, ulcers, should be closely monitored. A good number of people taking NSAIDs are also taking anti-ulcer meds at the same time. There is now a new class of drugs on the market known as "Cox-inhibitors" (Celebrex and Vioxx), which claim to have fewer side effects.

Over-the-counter medications such as aspirin, ibuprofen, and acetaminophen can also reduce inflammation. If medications don't work for your parent, there are also physical and occupational therapy (these guys help you figure out how to make daily-living tasks easier to perform) or even surgery to replace hip and knee joints.

Chronic Obstructive Pulmonary Disease (COPD)

COPD stands for chronic obstructive pulmonary (lung) disease. It's the umbrella term for emphysema and chronic bronchitis. Approximately 16.4 million Americans suffer from COPD, which is the fourth leading cause of death, claiming the lives of 100,360 Americans in 1996. Nearly 2 million Americans have emphysema, of which 55.5 percent are male and 44.5 percent are female. While more men suffer from the disease than do women, the condition is increasing among women. The major culprit in COPD is smoking. In emphysema, lung tissue breaks down and fills up with dead space. Stale air gets trapped in these spaces and prevents oxygen from getting exchanged. In bronchitis the bronchi produce excessive mucus because they are thickened and inflamed from scarring. Smoking and air pollution take credit for COPD. Frequent and long-lasting colds, deep coughs that bring up mucous, and breathlessness are sure signs.

There are a good number of treatments for these respiratory conditions that can prevent more damage. Check out your local American Lung Association and your parents' family doctor for treatment. In serious cases, your parents should be seen by a pulmonary (lung) specialist. And if they're smoking, help them to stop, using the "patch" or other method. Smoking with COPD is a lethal combination.

Sage Source

For more information about COPD, contact the American Lung Association, 1-800-586-4872; www.lungusa.org.

The Least You Need to Know

- Eighty-five percent of people affected by incontinence are women. Don't let your mom keep this a secret and resign herself to adult briefs—she can do something about it.

- Your parents should be seeing an eye doctor every year to be on the alert for diseases such as glaucoma, macular degeneration, cataracts, and diabetic retinopathy. Make sure an eye physician (ophthalmologist) is part of the team.

- Adult-onset diabetes affects one in four elderly over the age of 85 years. Your mom is more likely to get it than your dad.

- Osteoporosis causes millions of broken bones and 300,000 hip fractures every year, afflicting far more women than men. Daily calcium supplements can help prevent osteoporosis.

- If your parents are taking anti-inflammatory drugs for their arthritis like aspirin and NSAIDS, make sure their doctor is watching out for a major side affect—ulcers.

- A major culprit in COPD—the fourth leading cause of death—is smoking. If your mom or dad smoke, do all you can to help them to stop.

Chapter 4

Not-So-Normal Aging: The Mental Side

In This Chapter

- Why mental health problems are being missed among the elderly
- Alcohol abuse and the elderly
- Risk factors of depression and suicide
- Anxiety disorders
- Seeking help: who to see and what they can do
- How lifestyle changes can change your outlook

John Wayne never had a therapist. A guy like that just wouldn't go to one. Neither would Humphrey Bogart or Clark Gable. And then comes our generation, with Woody Allen's angst splattered all over the silver screen. You get the picture. Our parents' generation, despite our mom's devotion to Dr. Spock, views having a therapist as being pretty weak.

And that's too bad. Because as we age, we become more at risk for depression and other emotional problems that require more than just a shoulder to cry on. And the medical establishment seems to play into our parents' John Wayne bravado: Studies show that doctors are slow to pick up on depression and mental illness in older patients. They often don't go past "I'm doing fine" to explore whether or not your mom is adjusting to widowhood in a healthy manner or if your dad's extremely negative reaction to retirement is just a phase he's going through.

So, it's up to you to be sensitive to your parents' mental health. Chances are your parents aren't going to be gushing forth all of their emotional needs. You'll have to read between the lines and help them see that it's just as important to take care of their mental health as their physical health.

Why Your Parents' Mental Health Is at Risk

Your mom and dad may not have a history of mental health problems, but with all the physiological and life changes they experience as they age, they may indeed need the benefit of psychological services. Here are some of the more common factors that will tax your parents' mental health.

Changes in Sleep Patterns

Between 30 to 50 percent of the elderly experience chronic problems with sleep disturbance. We all know that wiped-out feeling we get from pulling an all-nighter. So you can imagine what this does to your mom or dad. In Chapter 2, "Getting to Know a Different Body," we went over the sleep changes that your parents can normally expect and how to get a good night's sleep. But if Dad is clearly having problems sleeping, causing him to be irritable and fatigued throughout the day, he should see a doctor. Sleep deprivation is a known contributor to depression. Problems of getting a good night's sleep can also be a symptom of a host of medical problems. So heed the warning.

Sage Source

The *Merck Manual of Geriatrics* is a classic medical reference book on identifying, understanding, and treating conditions that affect the elderly. You can now get it for free on the Internet. Just go to www.merck.com. You'll also find the *Merck Manual Home Edition* online for all of your family members.

Medications

Pills might solve one problem but they can contribute to depression. Sleep medications (hypnotics) often list depression as a possible side effect. Pills for arthritis, ulcers, heart problems, and high blood pressure can also contribute to depression. Be sure to read the fine print about various side effects of medications that your parent takes. If your parent is acting depressed and depression is listed as part of the drug manufacturer's warning, advise your parent's prescribing doctor of your mom's change in behavior.

Fears

Roosevelt said it best: "The only thing we have to fear is fear itself." The trouble is, your parents might have quite a few fears quietly eating away at them. Fears of having a catastrophic illness like a stroke, of being placed in a nursing home, of losing all of their life savings, of being abandoned, of being a burden to you, of you taking them out of their home and having them live with you, of dying … all take their toll on mental health. While most people have some level of fear in these areas, it's how they cope with the fear and measure it against reality that makes the difference between a healthy adjustment to aging and one that's in trouble.

These fears can also get in the way of telling you the truth about physical problems. A dear friend of mine in her 80s has yet to tell her son that she fell in the bathroom, cutting her head. She doesn't know how long she lay unconscious from the fall. It did propel her, however, to decide it was time for assisted living. But she *feared* if she told her son, he would have immediately intervened insisting she sell the house and move in with him.

Senior Alert

You might be surprised at the role television plays in your parents' fears. Many seniors spend a great deal of time watching daytime television and CNN. With the likes of talk show hosts Jerry Springer and Jenny Jones exposing the unraveling of civil society, along with events like school shootings on CNN, older people may see the world as a very frightening place, especially if they are relatively homebound and television becomes the prism from which they view the world.

Multiple Losses

There are some gains in aging: Respect in one's community and profession, wisdom, freedom from responsibilities, and the joys of grandparenting are a few. But there are also many losses: The loss of a job for many men can mean a loss of self-esteem and the network of friends from the office. Women also experience this loss; however, they seem to have a greater network of friends to more easily make the transition from work to retirement. If your dad's whole identity was his work, he might find retirement a disaster, feeling like he isn't capable of anything, isn't important, and life has no meaning. Loss of income and living on a restricted income can be interpreted as a loss of power. To exert a sense of power, your dad may adamantly insist on picking up the tab for dinner even though he can't afford it. Loss of strength loudly proclaimed by the need for a cane, a hearing aid, a wheel chair, and/or glasses is always a hit on one's ego.

As we discussed in Chapter 2, hearing loss, for example, can also cause your dad to become isolated, angry, and irritable at not understanding people, and even a bit paranoid that people are quietly talking about him. And then, of course, there's the loss of what our youth-adoring culture views as attractive: Rather than view gray hairs and wrinkles as something we've earned, we do everything to hide or remove them. If your mom or dad has a number of these losses hitting at the same time or in fast succession, don't assume they'll naturally get through it like they always have.

Alcohol

Alcohol not only places wear and tear on vital organs, it wreaks havoc with your parents' mental health. Psychological problems of denial, changes in mood, abusiveness, and impairment quickly join the fray. That liquor bottle can cause a vicious cycle. Your dad might be feeling down and take a drink to "soothe the pain." He'll drown it out for a short period of time and then feel the worse for it. He might also think that it will help him sleep better. But it will actually work against him. He'll also find that his aging body is more sensitive to the affects of alcohol than when he was younger. Studies show that a 60-year-old has a 20 percent *higher* blood-alcohol level than a 20-year-old drinking the *same* amount of alcohol.

Throw into the mix medications and decreased food intake, your dad, who might not have had a problem with alcohol abuse before, can certainly have one now. Your parents need to know how alcohol will affect them differently from their younger days.

Geri-Fact

In a recent study supported by the Agency for Health Care Policy and Research, one in 10 primary care patients 60 years of age and older had current evidence of alcoholism. Yet, fewer than half had diagnostic information picking up the disease in their medical records. Older alcoholic patients were more likely to be hospitalized and die than nonalcoholic patients.

The National Institute on Aging reports that drinking problems can be either chronic or situational. Chronic abusers have been heavy drinkers for years, while situational drinkers start drinking due to events such as the death of a spouse, retirement, or problems with sleeping or pain. Your mom might have been a teetotaler all of her life but now finds herself having a few nightcaps for a good night's sleep, then a few drinks to get through the day because of arthritis pain, and then a few more to cope with your dad's death. Numerous studies and reports reveal that alcoholism is often left undetected among the elderly. Primary care physicians don't probe, and patients don't tell. Adult children either feel it's too late to do something about Dad's chronic drinking or they think Mom's symptoms of confusion, forgetfulness, and frequent falls are due to old age and have nothing to do with the empty liquor bottles piling up in the recycle bin.

According to the National Council on Alcoholism and Drug Dependence, "Alcoholism is a primary, chronic disease with genetic, psychosocial, and environmental factors influencing its development and manifestations. The disease is often progressive and fatal. It is characterized by continuous or periodic: impaired control over drinking, preoccupation with the drug alcohol, use of alcohol despite adverse consequences, and distortions in thinking, most notably denial."

If your parent answers yes to any one of the following (known as the **CAGE** questionnaire), then he or she is symptomatic of alcoholism:

- Have you ever felt you should **C**ut down on your drinking?
- Have people **A**nnoyed you by criticizing your drinking?
- Have you ever felt bad or **G**uilty about your drinking?
- Have you ever had a drink first thing in the morning to steady your nerves or get rid of a hangover (**E**ye-opener)?

Senior Alert

If your parent has had an alcohol abuse problem and is admitted to a nursing home, alert the medical staff and nurses at admission. Don't try to hide the fact or think that now Dad will finally lick this problem. Withdrawal poses serious medical complications that must be treated by a physician. They need to know.

When It's More Than Just the Blues

Depression is the most common mental health problem of older people, yet it is often overlooked as a clinical disorder with serious complications. Grieving over the death of a friend, relative, or spouse can certainly leave your mom and dad feeling depressed. That's normal and healthy. But much of our society believes that depression goes hand-in-hand with old age. They think that with all of the losses older people go through, the aches and pains that they have, and the closer they get to dying—they *should* be depressed. It's natural to be depressed when you're old. Wrong! Many older people, in fact, have reached a point in life where they feel fulfilled, at peace with themselves, and glad to be out of the wear and tear of raising kids and climbing the career ladder.

Sage Source

For more information, contact the National Council on Alcoholism and Drug Dependence Hopeline (1-800-622-2255 or www.ncadd. org); Alcoholics Anonymous (212-870-3400 or www.alcoholics-anonymous.org); National Clearinghouse for Alcohol and Drug Information (1-800-729-6686 or www.health.org); or Al-Anon Family Groups, Inc. (1-888-4AL-ANON or www.al-anon. alateen.org).

Even though the good news is that it's not normal for your parents to be depressed, the bad news is if they are depressed, it's likely to be ignored. Doctors and family members simply don't pick up on it partly because—you guessed it—everybody thinks it's an age thing. The challenge for you—and this is a tough one—is to know when it's not just the blues.

What Is Depression?

Depression is an illness of intense sadness that interferes with the ability to function, feel pleasure, or maintain interest. Researchers have discovered that biochemical imbalances in the brain go hand in hand with depression. It may follow a recent loss or other sad event but the intensity of responding to the event and the duration persists far beyond what is healthy. The illness isn't just psychological. Counseling alone won't bring someone out of it, nor will a good talking to as in "Mom, you've just got to snap yourself out of this." She can't talk away the biochemical changes in her body.

Depression is complicated. Scientists aren't sure what triggers it, but they do know it can be linked to genetics, loss, fear of illness and death, stress, hormonal changes, isolation, physical illness, and medications. Women are twice as likely as men to be depressed, often responding to adversity by withdrawing or blaming themselves. Female hormonal changes are also suspected of making women more vulnerable.

Senior Alert

The National Institute of Mental Health (NIMH) estimates that although about one in five people over 60 suffers from levels of depression that require medical intervention, most receive no treatment of any kind.

Silver Lining

The National Institute of Mental Health reports that a combination of psychotherapy and medications has an 80 percent success rate in helping older adults beat depression.

So What Can You Do?

Check out the following list for the signs of depression. If you suspect your mom is depressed, try talking to her about bringing this up with her primary or family physician. Ask her to describe *what* she's feeling. Acknowledge that you know she just hasn't been herself and that depression can take on a life of its own. Let her know that you understand that she isn't controlling what she feels. You know that she's not just sitting around feeling sorry for herself. Reassure her that there are things that can be done, but she'll need a doctor to sort things out.

Symptoms of Clinical Depression (from the U.S. Department of Health and Human Services)

1. Persistent sadness, anxiety, or empty mood

2. Loss of interest or pleasure in ordinary activities, family, or friends

3. Decreased energy, listlessness, fatigue, feeling "slowed down" especially in the morning

4. Sleep problems and changes in sleep patterns (can't get to sleep, over-sleeping, waking up too early)

5. Eating problems and changes in eating patterns or foods consumed (weight loss or gain, gain or loss in appetite)

6. Difficulty concentrating, remembering, or making decisions

7. Feelings of hopelessness or pessimism

8. Feelings of guilt, worthlessness, hopelessness or helplessness

9. Thoughts of suicide or death

10. Irritability

11. Excessive crying, sometimes without reason

12. Recurring aches and pains (headaches, backaches) that don't respond to treatment

It would be good if you can go to this doctor's appointment with your mom or at least talk to the doctor ahead of time. Don't, however, make this into some James Bond operation behind her back. You'll only be sending her the message that this is something shameful. Simply describe the symptoms as you would any other illness. Given her state of mind, however, she might need a little help in describing the symptoms and how they have affected her daily life. You also can be a good resource on how this is different from any past ways Mom has reacted to problems. Doctors often use standardized questionnaires and blood work to diagnose depression.

Can a Pill Fix It?

Now to make this even tougher, here's an adage to keep in mind, "The cure can be worse than the disease." Antidepressant drugs can be great but they should not be dispensed until a differential diagnosis (figuring out what's really wrong) has been made. Just giving out an antidepressant without knowing the underlying cause can mask a serious health problem that will only get worse. Studies have shown that far too many elderly are given a pill rather than offered psychotherapy or other mental health services.

These drugs are also very powerful and it takes time to get the dosing just right—especially among the elderly. Their body's drug absorption rate is different from the younger subjects that the drug companies tested before it was made available to the general public. A geriatric psychiatrist is the best prepared physician to figure out what is best for your mom. The right medication with the correct dosage can do wonders but be sure to monitor your parent's reaction to the drug very carefully!

The National Institute of Mental Health's depression cue card.

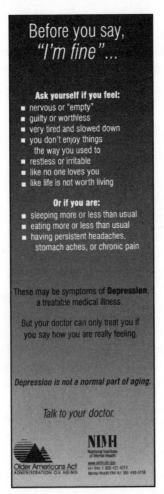

Suicide

Severe depression left unchecked can result in suicide. Your dad's age group (65 years plus) has the highest suicide rate of any age group in the country! White males over

85 years of age are at greatest risk. In the midst of writing this book, a dear friend's Dad took his life. He had never had a history of depression or mental illness. He was a hard worker, loved his family, and didn't have any money problems. But a complication during back surgery left him with even more physical problems, another surgery, and a tremendous amount of pain. His last comment from his doctor's appointment was "I just wish they could just give me some hope." He ended his life days later with a loving note to his family assuring them it had nothing to do with them. He just couldn't live with the pain and despair one day longer. My friend's dad fit the pattern—a recent study has shown that 40 percent of elderly suicide victims saw their primary physician within one week of committing suicide, and 70 percent within the month! The bottom line? Even the doctors aren't picking up on our parents' suicidal state of mind.

If your mom or dad has symptoms of depression, don't simply look the other way thinking they'll get past it without any help. Share with them the NIMH depression cue card shown earlier. Urge them to seek help from their primary care physician or a mental health specialist.

Senior Alert

Going back and forth between different antidepressants can pose serious problems for your parent. Don't let insurance companies or pharmacists, who have been given an incentive by drug companies, switch your parent's medications without your parent, you, and the doctor knowing the full ramifications of what the change in medication can mean.

Geri-Fact

White males 85 years and over commit suicide at six times the national rate! Making up 13 percent of the U.S. population, individuals 65 years and over disproportionately account for 20 percent of all suicides.

Anxiety Disorders

Ever have your 17-year-old tell you to *chill out* or accuse you of worrying too much? It's pretty hard not to be an anxious parent as your teenager walks out the door with keys in hand. If you didn't worry, something would be wrong. But if your dad appears to be excessively worried about the future, feels nervous tension, or has become very fearful, he might be experiencing an anxiety disorder. About one in 10 adults over 55 years of age has this condition to a point where medical help is needed to get over it. You need a professional to figure out if this is related to a physical problem or is psychological. Anti-anxiety drugs must be prescribed very carefully and for a very short period of time. Be very cautious of the class of drugs known as benzodiazepines: They tend to become habit forming, and are known to cause respiratory problems, depression, and psychomotor impairment that can turn your dad into a terrible driver, make him confused, and impair his memory.

Seeking Help

Make sure you're working with a doctor who fully appreciates mental health problems among the elderly and is up on a variety of treatments from counseling to drug therapy and lifestyle changes including nutrition and exercise, along with other alternative medicine responses. You also want a physician who will spend the time to do a thorough investigation into what is causing your mom's depression. It could be something as simple as a side effect from one of the many drugs she is taking. Or it could be a thyroid problem. Or it could be … you get the point.

Sage Source

For more information, contact the National Institute of Mental Health's Depression Awareness and Treatment Program (1-800-421-4211 or www.nimh.nih.gov) or the National Foundation for Depressive Illness (1-800-248-4381 or www.depression.org).

Silver Lining

For preventing and beating depression through nutrition and vitamins for your parents and yourself, take a look at *The Complete Idiot's Guide for Living Longer and Healthier*, by Dr. Allan Magaziner (Alpha Books, 1999).

A geriatric psychiatrist—a physician who specializes in the mental health, diseases and treatment of the elderly—can be extremely helpful in diagnosing what's wrong. If you live in an area where none are readily available, look for a physician who has certification in geriatrics. Many hospitals now offer geriatric specialty clinics that have psychologists and social workers who are specially trained in this field.

There are a number of things the physician might prescribe: antidepressant drugs (it takes two to three months for these to become fully effective) usually along with psychotherapy, relaxation exercises, and lifestyle changes that include nutrition and exercise.

The physician will probably measure how your parent thinks, known as cognitive functioning, to see if his or her mental health problem is due to physical changes in the brain. One of the most common mini-mental-status exams you'll hear about is the Folstein, which measures memory and the ability to calculate, follow instructions, and comprehend. Your parent will also be given questionnaires (Beck Depression Inventory, for example) to pick up symptoms of depression. Blood work will also be ordered to pick up biochemical and hormonal changes.

A treatment of last resort in extreme cases of depression is electroconvulsive (ECT) therapy. In this procedure the patient is given an anesthetic and muscle relaxant. Electric pulses are sent through the temple by way of a padded electrode. A minor brain seizure is induced. Yes, this sounds pretty rough but it has proven to be successful and at times, life-saving; however, it is not usually recommended for someone with dementia.

Lifestyle Changes: Good for the Mind

In addition to any of the treatments offered to help your parent cope with his or her mental health problem, good nutrition, vitamins, exercise, and an active social life should always be part of the plan. Research has shown that one in four people with depression are deficient in some form of B vitamin. Sugar is another known culprit offering a quick fix for feeling "up" but then throwing your mood back down into the dumps an hour later. Since depression is a biochemical illness there's nothing like exercise to get your brain producing endorphins to raise your mood level. Don't underestimate how remaining active, being involved, and feeling needed can ward off depression. If your mom or dad is physically capable of being active, there are a zillion ways to volunteer. Call your local religious group, senior center, YWCA, local Girls or Boys Club, school, or local AARP chapter for opportunities.

The Least You Need to Know

- Depression is one of the most common mental health problems of the elderly and much of the time it isn't even diagnosed or treated. Yet, with treatment, 80 percent of the elderly with depression recover.

- Older men have the highest suicide rate of any age group in the country—don't let your dad's depression go unchecked.

- Alcohol mixed with depression, medications, and a change in physiology can create a dangerous mix for your parents.

- The class of drugs known as benzodiazepines often used for sleeping and anxiety problems can cause other side affects and become addictive. Make sure your doctor is aware of any adverse reactions that your parent may have to these drugs.

- A healthy lifestyle of exercise, nutrition, vitamins, and remaining socially active can go a long way toward staying mentally fit.

Chapter 5

Brain Attacks (Strokes) and Heart Attacks

In This Chapter

- Brain attack and heart attack basics
- Know the warning signs
- Understanding the lingo
- What you can do to reduce the risks
- Four conditions that can lead to heart attacks

The one thing that my dad fears most is a stroke. The last thing he wants is to be like Oscar, a buddy who lived in the fast lane but ended his days on the sidelines strapped to a wheelchair after a debilitating stroke. The fact that my dad's father had a stroke increases his odds of having one himself. My mom fears cancer. Her dad died of it and so did far too many friends. A dear friend of mine, a retired nursing home administrator, fears Alzheimer's. All of them think about heart attacks.

The big four—strokes, heart attacks, Alzheimer's disease, and cancer—are what most older people fear. They are also what adult children fear most for their parents. Even though great strides have been and are being made in treating these conditions, they can be catastrophic. For good reason: Strokes, heart attacks, and cancer are the leading causes of death among older people in this country.

In this chapter, we'll take a look at the attackers: brain attacks and heart attacks. In the next chapter we'll cover Alzheimer's disease and cancer.

Brain Attacks (Strokes)

The "in" term these days for strokes is brain attack. Ever wonder who makes these decisions? But the new term actually makes more sense. Just as a heart attack results in less blood and oxygen getting to the heart, so it is with a stroke, which cuts off blood supply from part of the brain. An artery might be clogged or a vessel tears, leaking the blood before and/or after it reaches the brain. *How many* brain cells are damaged and *where* those cells are located depends on what part of the brain didn't receive its blood supply.

Given the fact that the human brain has more functions than Carter has liver pills, and that any part can get a "sorry, we can't deliver" message, the ways in which strokes affect people are all over the map. A whole side can be paralyzed (usually the right), or just one part of the body such as an arm. Some people experience behavioral changes while some can't swallow, speak, write, or urinate. Even if the stroke was mild, if it affected a part of the brain that controls a major function, the result can be devastating.

Brain Attack Lingo

If your parent suffers a stroke, there are a number of terms you'll hear and there are different kinds of strokes. Here's what you ought to know.

Senior Alert

A major study of 30,000 older people who suffered a stroke showed that patients who were seen by a neurologist within the first 72 hours had a much better recovery and survival rate than those who did not. Be sure to ask that a neurologist examine your parent right away.

TIA

TIA stands for transient ischemic (pronounced *iss-chemic*) attack. You may hear it referred to as a "mini-stroke," but your doctor will probably call it a TIA. It comes on suddenly and usually lasts from two to 30 minutes. There is a temporary deficiency in the brain's blood supply. The symptoms are similar to a stroke but they are temporary and reversible. So your dad might get dizzy, might not be able to see, and might experience slurred speech for about three minutes and then return back to normal. *This is a warning sign.* Just because a TIA appeared out of the clear blue sky and then disappeared doesn't mean he's in the clear. About one third of all strokes are preceded by a TIA and about half will hit within the year. So make sure your dad sees a doctor. There are plenty of ways to prevent a stroke. Don't let it go!

Ischemic Stroke

With an ischemic stroke, an artery carrying blood to the brain is blocked, usually by fatty material. The lack of blood and oxygen damages the part of the brain that didn't get the goods—blood and oxygen.

Hemorrhagic Stroke

In this instance, the blood and oxygen makes its destination to the brain, however, the vessel carrying it bursts and leaks blood into the brain destroying brain cells in its wake. A stroke caused by hemorrhaging inside the brain is considered more dangerous and is involved in about 17 percent of stroke cases. Your doctor might group ischemic and hemorrhagic strokes together and refer to them as a cerebrovascular accident.

Strokes are America's number three killer, right after heart attacks and cancer. You and your parents should be aware of the symptoms. This is definitely the time to call 911.

The American Heart Association lists the following stroke signals:

- Sudden weakness or numbness of the face, arm, and leg on one side of the body
- Sudden confusion, trouble speaking or understanding
- Dimness or loss of vision, particularly in one eye
- Sudden trouble walking, dizziness, loss of balance or coordination
- Sudden severe headache with no known cause

The Stroke Forecast

If your parent has a stroke, you'll learn that the first two days are crucial for your parent's recovery. It's a tough wait-and-see vigil until you know the extent of the damage. The doctor might order a *CT scan* or a *MRI* to help him or her pinpoint the cause of the stroke.

The good news is that many people recover from their strokes and can resume a normal life. For others, it will be a tougher recovery period and will involve some intensive rehabilitation. Your parent will need a lot of support and you should be on guard for depression. Regretfully, about 20 percent of the people who have strokes will die, never leaving the hospital. Those in their 80s and 90s are especially vulnerable.

Geri-Fact

A **CT** (Computed Tomography) **scan** is a computer-enhanced x-ray study that detects structural abnormalities on any part of the body. A **MRI** (Magnetic Resonance Imaging) is a magnetic imaging test that detects structural abnormalities on any part of the body.

If your mom or dad has high blood pressure, definitely make sure he or she monitors it. I'll never forget the day the ambulance came to rescue our dear friend and neighbor. He'd suffered a debilitating stroke from which it took two years to recover. He hadn't been taking his blood pressure medicine.

Preventing Strokes

Your parent can do more to prevent a stroke than modern medical technology can do. According to the National Institutes of Health, the most treatable conditions linked to stroke are:

- **High blood pressure.** A well-balanced diet, healthy weight, and exercise are a sure formula to control high blood pressure. Medications can also control it. *Bottom line: Treat it.*

- **Cigarette smoking.** Plenty of evidence has shown that cigarette smoking highly increases risk for stroke. *Bottom line: Quit.*

- **Diabetes.** Complications from diabetes contribute to strokes. *Bottom line: Control the diabetes to reduce the chance of strokes.*

- **Heart disease.** Heart disease creates a friendly environment for strokes. Pills like aspirin can prevent clotting. *Bottom line: Manage your heart disease to ward off strokes.*

Sage Source

The National Institute of Neurological Disorders and Stroke has a top-notch Web site describing brain attacks and prevention strategies. Visit them at www.ninds.nih.gov. The National Stroke Association offers an excellent Web site (www.stroke.org) for stroke victims and their families. You can also track down stroke support groups near you from the site. Or you can call them at 1-800-STROKES.

Probably, the greatest barrier you'll face with changing your dad's (or mom's) lifestyle is the belief that he's too old to make a difference to his body. Or he'll contend that since the damage is already done, what's the point in changing? He needs to be convinced that, in fact, more damage can be done if he does nothing. And on the bright side, he can get better and even feel younger with a body given good nutrition, exercise, and a smoke-free environment.

Heart Attacks

Everyday in this country, over 1,300 people have a fatal heart attack. Four out of five victims are over 65 years old. To say this is an "age thing" is an understatement. But guess what? Even though heart disease is common among older people, it isn't because old hearts just give out like your car's motor.

It's because of what your mom and dad have done to their hearts—the smoking, the fatty foods clogging the arteries, the extra weight, the lack of exercise, and high blood pressure going unchecked—that will do their hearts in. The area that they can't control—a family history of heart disease—requires they be all the more vigilant about what they *can* control.

Parents in the Driver's Seat

You'll be fighting against old stereotypes and outdated medical opinions when you try convincing your parents that they, more than anyone else, can stave off a heart attack.

Just 15 years ago, the medical community thought that the cardiovascular system of older people just gave out with the wear and tear of normal aging. But along came this mega, 25-year study—the Baltimore Longitudinal Study on Aging by the National Institutes of Health. It was quite a shocker when they discovered that the older guy's hearts were pumping blood practically the same way as the young studs in the sample study. It wasn't *normal* aging, after all.

Senior Alert

Who's at risk for heart attacks?

- Parents who are smokers
- Overweight parents
- Parents with high blood pressure
- Parents with high cholesterol
- Diabetic parents
- Stressed-out parents (You better not be the cause!)
- "Couch potato" parents
- Parents with heart disease in the family tree

The Big Four "Widow Makers"

I can still see my dad's cardiologist (a doctor who specializes in treating the heart) pointing to an x-ray of Dad's clogged artery saying, "This is the one we call the widow maker." Lucky, for my dad his doctor tracked down the cause of his shortness of breath and unclogged his artery. There are four leading conditions that make your parents susceptible to heart attacks. Here's a nutshell explanation of each, with some tips on how your mom and dad can keep clear of these widow makers.

High Blood Pressure

Of all things that will put your parent at risk—high blood pressure is the "big one." It's also the one they can do something about. Imagine your garden hose hooked up to a fire truck. The pressure shooting through the hose would wear it thin in no time. Now imagine a small pump at the end of the hose trying to redirect the high-pressured water through other small hoses. Any bets on how long the pump can handle the pressure? In a less dramatic way, this is what high blood pressure does to your parent's heart. It's the continuous, high-pressured rush of blood flowing through blood vessel walls (hose-like arteries and veins) that wear them down to a point where they can tear or leak.

Geri-Fact

Blood pressure readings measure the force of blood coursing through your arteries. There are two numbers. Mine usually comes in at 110/80 (unless I've just read my teenage son's report card). The first number is the systolic blood pressure. It reads the force of the blood pressing up against the arteries in the arm with the blood pressure cuff on. The second or bottom number (diastolic) reads the pressure that remains in the arteries when the heart is relaxed. High numbers aren't good: consistently hitting 160 on the systolic is a sure sign to get to the doctor. Check with your doctor on what's considered high for your parent's age and weight.

Just about every drug store and even grocery stores have one of those cool machines where for a few quarters your mom can stick her arm in a tube and get a digital blood pressure reading. However, these machines may not be reliable, so if the reading is unusually high, follow it up with a reading from your family doctor. A blood pressure cuff also makes a great gift if your parent is homebound. Ask your family doctor or medical supply store if they can recommend a good, reliable brand for home use. Bottom line? There's no excuse for not knowing your blood pressure.

Reducing salt can bring down and control your high blood pressure. I'm not just talking about the table salt you sprinkle on your food. You'd be shocked at the salt (or sodium) content in many packaged or processed foods. Controlling weight, managing stress, and taking medications can also bring down the pressure levels. Diuretics are commonly prescribed because they take out salt and water from the circulatory system and send them off to the urinary system. Any medication has to be closely monitored by a physician so that other conditions your parent has aren't adversely affected. No matter what, a salty diet has to go and blood pressure checks should become routine. African-American families, especially, should be on high alert for high blood pressure because your parents are more likely than others to have high blood pressure.

Cholesterol

Let's go back to our garden hose example for a moment. Imagine fatty, sticky stuff stuck to the inside of the hose. There you are with your Martha Stewart garden gloves trying to water your prized red geraniums. A pathetic stream of water dribbles out. Cholesterol is the fatty sticky stuff stuck to your mom's blood vessels. When this stuff reaches a level that actually clogs the vessels, it's given a name: atherosclerosis. Cholesterol readings can tell your mom how much of this stuff is in her system. Your mom is at more risk of this if she smokes, has high blood pressure or diabetes, or is obese. If that's the case, it doesn't hurt to have her cholesterol checked once a year. If your mom's vessels get too clogged, that pathetic stream will cause real havoc with her heart.

To reduce the risk of artherosclerosis a low cholesterol diet is the way to go. But don't go over the top on your mom. Changing lifelong food habits is tough. She's been slowly building up the fatty sticky stuff over a lifetime. The deal is to get her to cut down on fats one step at a time. Most experts think that no more than 30 percent of our calories should come from fats. Today, your mom can easily determine how much fat she's getting by checking out the fat breakdown on the packaging of food products.

Want to practice what you preach? Reduce your *own* fat intake. According to the American Heart Association, there are two kinds of cholesterol:

- The "good" kind is called high-density lipoprotein (HDL). Your body makes HDL on its own for your protection. It's believed to actually carry cholesterol away from artery walls.

- "Bad" cholesterol, known as low-density lipoprotein (LDL), clogs the arteries and increases your risk for heart attacks.

Check out the American Heart Association's Web site at www.americanheart.org for all kinds of cholesterol information, diets, and treatments.

Angina

Last Christmas my dad went upstairs to haul out the annual Christmas tree. By the time he got back downstairs he stopped. My sister, a nurse, asked what he was doing. "I'm taking a break." My dad, who ran a dairy and still plows snow on his tractor at age 80, *never* takes a break. He finally confessed that he was feeling chest pains. Under the interrogation of my sister (trust me, it was an interrogation) he admitted to feeling chest pains every time he exerted himself. She knew he was experiencing angina, temporary chest pains or a sensation of pressure when the heart muscle isn't receiving enough oxygen.

Off to the doctor he went. And sure enough, he had a great deal of blockage in a major artery. He now has a stent (a small device that holds a narrowed coronary artery open). He's feeling much better. Good thing my sister caught on. My dad figured it was just old age. He thinks complaining is for wimps. Plenty of Dads think this way, so you really need to probe them for information. Maybe even take them to the mall and see how they do trying to keep up with you at a brisk walk.

Classic angina symptoms can consist of chest pains, indigestion, shortness of breath, and an odd ache around the neck that spreads to the jaw, throat, shoulder, back, or arms. *Always* get these symptoms checked out if either of your parents experience any one of them. It's a warning. And in my dad's case it was a blessing. Tests to determine what's really going on range from an EKG (electrocardiogram), stress tests, scans, and echocardiograms. If any of these tests turn up something, the doctor might recommend that your dad have a *catheterization*.

Geri-Fact

Cholesterol hides out in animal products: meat, poultry, seafood, organ meats, eggs, and dairy products such as butter and cheese. One egg yolk will just about blow one day's healthy limit of cholesterol.

Geri-Fact

During a **catheterization,** a cardiologist inserts a thin tube into a vein or artery. Using dye and an x-ray machine, the doctor can see on a monitor exactly where and how much blockage the patient has. The doctor can even determine how well the blood flows through the blood vessels.

If the doctor finds that there is a blockage of an artery or vein, he or she can either insert a tiny balloon to open up the vessel, put in a stent to keep the vessel open, or bypass the blocked vessel by detouring the unblocked vessels to the heart. There are also many medications that can help. Whatever you do, take the time to do some research. New advances are being made every day, so be sure to stay current.

Sage Source

The American Heart Association (www.americanheart.org) offers a wealth of information and links to other helpful sites. If you want to go to one Web site to get all of your information on heart disease, this is it. There's helpful information on strokes, too. Contact the American Heart Association, 7272 Greenville Avenue, Dallas, TX 75231; 1-800-242-1793. The National Heart, Lung, and Blood Institutes (www.nhlbi.nih.gov) also offers another good site. They can be reached at P.O. Box 30105, Bethesda, MD 20284; 301-251-1222.

Congestive Heart Failure (CHF)

If your mom or dad is given this diagnosis, the heart muscle itself is damaged. The damaged muscle slows down the heart's blood flow. Blood backs up either into the lungs or in the veins. In either case, it causes fluid congestion in the tissues. The goal? Damage control. Early intervention is key.

With congestive heart failure your dad might experience fatigue, shortness of breath, a hacking cough, waking up in the middle of the night feeling like he's suffocating, sudden weight gain of two to four pounds in a couple of days, swelling in the ankles, legs, or arms, and a rapid heart beat. Again, no fooling around. You and your dad are off to the cardiologist.

Chances are the doctor will prescribe some medication to keep the damaged heart from failing on the job. CHF is not a death sentence. The drugs Dad will take must be monitored very closely—no self-medicating. He must take the correct dosage. A healthy heart diet is definitely in order, too. The American Heart Association Web site offers healthy heart diets and a wealth of other resources on eating well.

New research has found that women have a higher heart attack death rate than men, more complications during hospitalizations for a heart attack, and different types of heart attacks than men. Women have a higher proportion of unstable angina—severe chest pains with no permanent clot. Older women with diabetes and high blood pressure are at greatest risk of dying from heart attacks; younger women (under 50 years) are twice as likely to die of a heart attack than their male counterparts. Don't make the mistake of thinking that heart attacks are a "guy thing." Look out for your mom, too.

The Most Common Heart Attack Warning Signs
(from the American Heart Association)

- Uncomfortable feeling of pressure, fullness, squeezing, or pain in the center of the chest lasting more than a few minutes
- Pain spreading to the shoulders, neck, or arms
- Chest discomfort with lightheadedness, fainting, sweating, nausea, or shortness of breath
- Atypical chest, stomach, or abdominal pain
- Nausea or dizziness
- Shortness of breath and difficulty breathing
- Unexplained anxiety, weakness, or fatigue
- Palpitations, cold sweat, or paleness

The Least You Need to Know

- High blood pressure is the leading and most preventable cause of brain attacks (strokes).

- Heart attacks and strokes, respectively, are the first and third leading killers among the elderly.

- Your parents' lifestyles contribute more to heart attacks than old age: Quit smoking and control cholesterol, diabetes, and blood pressure.

- Your mom or dad can recover from a stroke; the first 72 hours are vital for a good prognosis. Heed the warning of mini-strokes.

- Most people report feeling "like new again" following bypass surgery or other procedures that clean or open clogged arteries.

Chapter 6

Alzheimer's Disease and Cancer

In This Chapter

- The difference between dementia and forgetfulness
- Dementia warning signs and what to do
- The stages of Alzheimer's disease
- When the diagnosis is cancer: what to ask
- Cancer basics
- Tracking down cancer treatment

My teenagers forget everything. I drop them off at school and an hour later I get a desperate call, "Please, Mom, I forgot my paper, this is life and death. For real! *Please,* I've got to have it by fourth period!" I know I'm not the only parent getting these calls. Forgetfulness seems to go with the territory with teens. We chalk it up to hormones.

But when my 80-year-old dad starts forgetting the names of old friends, or Mom forgets my brother's phone number that she's been dialing for years ... they worry. And so do we. Without saying it, everyone's secretly wondering, "Could this be the first sign of Alzheimer's?"

Alzheimer's: Just How Common Is It?

Should my dad be *this* worried? Let's try to put this in perspective. About four million people have Alzheimer's disease in this country. According to the National Institutes of Health, about 3 percent of people between the ages of 65 and 74 have Alzheimer's. This incidence dramatically increases with advancing age; nearly half of the population over 85 years has the disease. Most people live an average of eight to 10 years from the onset of symptoms. Yes, it is something to be on guard for, especially as your parents enter their mid-80s, but it certainly isn't something that every older person has to fear lurking around the corner.

Dementia and Alzheimer's Disease

Dementia is actually an umbrella term (literally meaning "without mind") that refers to the progressive loss of thinking, judgment, ability to focus, and ability to learn. More than half of the dementia cases are caused by Alzheimer's, a disease named after German physician Alois Alzheimer who discovered it back in 1906. No one is exactly sure what causes Alzheimer's, but genetic factors are definitely in the mix.

The second leading cause of dementia is multi-infarct dementia caused by the death of brain cells due to mini-strokes that block blood supply. These small, successive strokes often go unnoticed as they chip away at the brain. People with high blood pressure and diabetes are at considerable risk for this type of dementia.

Sage Source

The Alzheimer's Association is an excellent organization that offers a wide range of information and support services. The have a nationwide network of chapters that hold monthly support meetings. Visit their Web site at www.alz.org to find a chapter near you, receive medical information, link to great resources, get expert advice online, and obtain a caregiver guide; or call them at 1-800-272-3900.

The Warning Signs

Everybody gets distracted. Everybody forgets a name, and everybody has misplaced their keys at one time or another. And some of us have even forgotten where we parked the car. So if all this is normal, how do you know when forgetfulness slides into the world of dementia?

The Alzheimer's Association has developed a list of the top 10 warning signs of Alzheimer's. If Mom or Dad experiences several of these symptoms, it's time to get him or her to a doctor. One way you can be very helpful when you've scheduled your parent for a checkup for dementia is to make a copy of this list and write up the behaviors exhibited by your parent under each symptom. The behaviors that you cite should not be typical life-long behaviors of your mom or dad. (My kids, for instance, certainly wouldn't list losing car keys as a sign for me!)

The Top 10 Warning Signs of Alzheimer's Disease (from the Alzheimer's Association)

1. **Memory loss affecting job skills.** Frequently forgets assignments, colleague's names; appears confused for no reason.

2. **Difficulty performing familiar tasks.** Easily distracted; forgets what he or she was doing or why. Might prepare a meal and then forget to serve it, or that he or she even made it.

3. **Problems with language.** Forgets simple words or substitutes inappropriate words; doesn't make sense.

4. **Disorientation to time and place.** May become lost on his or her own street; doesn't know where he or she is, how he or she got there, or how to get back home.

5. **Poor or decreased judgment.** Usually exhibited through wearing inappropriate clothing, or poor grooming. Forgets to wear a coat when it's cold; wears a bathrobe to the store.

6. **Problems with abstract thinking.** Exhibits trouble with numbers; can no longer make simple calculations.

7. **Misplaces things.** Not only loses things, but puts things in inappropriate places, such as putting a purse in the freezer or a wristwatch in a sugar bowl. Has no idea how the items got there.

8. **Mood and behavior changes.** Exhibits more rapid mood swings for no apparent reason.

9. **Changes in personality.** Dramatic change in personality; for example, someone who was easygoing now appears extremely uptight. Becoming suspicious and fearful are commonly reported.

10. **Loss of initiative.** Becomes extremely disinterested and uninvolved in areas that he or she used to enjoy.

If You Think Your Mom or Dad Has Dementia

How do you know for sure? The only way an absolute diagnosis can be made is through an autopsy where plaque, tangles, and abnormal proteins appear on the brain. Well, you're not about to get your dad tested this way! So how do doctors know?

Diagnosing Alzheimer's is really a process of elimination. The first step is for your dad's primary physician to rule out any reversible signs of dementia, such as a drug reaction that causes him to be confused. If that's not the case, he should be seen y a geriatrician or a neurologist (a doctor who specializes in the nervous system). A full workup takes two to three hours. The physician should listen to you and other family members describe changes in your dad's behavior.

The evaluation will include a Mini-Mental Status Exam which is a short test to determine your dad's ability to handle simple tasks, work with numbers, communicate, recall new and recent information, and process abstract thought. As a result, Dad will probably be asked to name the current President, count backwards, draw a familiar object, and complete a task with simple instructions. The evaluation can include a neurological exam; blood and urine tests to determine if he has a condition that can cause confusion such as a thyroid abnormality or vitamin B-12 deficiency; and various scans such as a CAT and MRI of the brain to identify damage from a stroke, seizure, or blood clot. The scan may also pick up the accumulation of spinal fluid. A spinal tap may be ordered if an infection or disease of the nervous system is suspected. And finally, a psychiatric consult is advised to identify possible causes of Dad's symptoms that might not be related to dementia such as depression.

Since there is no definite, proof-positive test to determine Alzheimer's, as can be done with cancer or diabetes, doctors rely on a battery of tests to rule everything else out. In 5 to 10 percent of the cases, the symptoms that appear to be dementia are caused by a condition that can be reversed. This might be a good point to use to convince Dad he should be evaluated. He may be trying to hide his symptoms for fear of Alzheimer's and refuse to see a doctor. Letting your dad know that there are a number of reasons that could account for what he is experiencing might alleviate his fears and encourage him to find out what's really wrong. Either way it turns out, he and you will be better for knowing the truth.

Sage Source

To receive the latest information on new treatments, track down clinical trials, or find a national Alzheimer's Disease Center near your parents, contact Alzheimer's Disease Education and Referral (ADEAR) at 1-800-438-4380. They also have a terrific Web site (www. alzheimers.org) that can connect you directly to the 29 national Alzheimer's disease centers throughout the United States. The site also keeps you posted on the results of the latest research.

Regretfully, there is no cure for dementia and Alzheimer's disease. If this is the diagnosis, you'll need to work closely with your parent's physician to monitor the effects of any medications your parent is taking. Drugs can help treat some of the symptoms and promising new drugs are being introduced every year. Gingko and vitamin E also have been reported to slow the progression of the disease for some people.

Be aware that psychotropic drugs (mind-altering) are very powerful. Figuring out the right dosage may take time and these drugs should never be mixed with alcohol. However, most of the care for someone with Alzheimer's is not medical. It involves a lot of love, support, and creative strategies to make life familiar and safe for your parent. For help on caring for someone with dementia, see Chapter 18, "Caring for Someone at Home: The Basics."

The Three Stages of Alzheimer's Disease

There are three basic stages that most people with Alzheimer's experience:

- During **Stage I** Dad has trouble remembering anything recent. He has a hard time concentrating, his speech may be slightly impaired, he has trouble thinking of the right word, he doesn't care about his personal grooming, abstract thinking is out of reach for him, and he easily gets upset, anxious, or angry. Other days he may be depressed.

- In **Stage II** Dad's behavior becomes much more extreme. His short-term memory is nearly gone, his coordination is poor, and he needs help getting dressed, eating, or bathing. Making decisions—even choosing what to wear—seem overwhelming. He becomes easily agitated and begins wandering or pacing back and forth. It's harder to understand him as his speech and language skills deteriorate. You may hear the same story repeatedly or he may repeat the same action almost incessantly. He can become outraged for no reason. His sleep cycles are disturbed and nighttime wandering is common.

- In **Stage III** Dad is in the final stages of the disease. Even his long-term memory has faded away, and he needs total care. What becomes most difficult for families is the paranoia Dad may experience, believing those around him are out to hurt him. His joints become rigid and his range of motion limited; eventually he becomes bedridden, unable to speak or feed himself. His immune system becomes dangerously weakened, leaving him vulnerable to pneumonia and other infections.

Not everyone experiences each of these behaviors, but it's important for you to know what to expect. Your dad doesn't love you any less if he forgets your name, can't recall his marriage, or lashes out at you. Most of the care for someone with Alzheimer's is not medical. It takes a lot of love and support. Join a support group to learn how to cope and make life better for your dad. Also, be sure to read Chapter 24, "Planning for Incapacity."

The Big "C": Cancer

I remember when I had a biopsy done on a mole. Two days later I answered the phone and the nurse said, "The doctor wants to speak to you." Alarm bells went off in my head. Hey, I was just expecting one of those postcards saying your tests came back negative, not a personal call. "Linda, there's good news and bad news." Never a good opening. I went for the bad news first. "Linda, you have malignant melanoma, and it spreads very fast. You need to see an internist right away to see if it has. I also want you to see a plastic surgeon for a wide excision of your back." It's amazing how you process this type of information. It really feels like hearing a verdict—only you missed the trial. It's also like an out-of-body experience. We went on to the good news: The cancer was a Stage II, meaning it hadn't progressed very far. He felt we had caught it in time. I had the surgery and a battery of tests; five years later I'm in the clear.

Your Parent's View

I share this with you because, although we all dread cancer, it's estimated that 40 percent of the adults diagnosed with cancer do survive. Every year, as a result of aggressive cancer research, new methods to stave off the progression of cancer are being discovered. Your parents, however, come from a generation where cancer wasn't talked about. They might have felt ashamed if their parents had it so they didn't tell their friends. It was common for families to engage in a conspiracy of silence, believing it was in the cancer victim's best interest not to know he or she had cancer.

Times have changed dramatically; however, your mom and dad's views might still be back in the 1950s. They might not tell you or their doctor that they have symptoms for fear of finding out that they have cancer. Just as it seemed as if I was given a verdict, they think that it's a death sentence, given what they saw when they were young adults. They're trapped thinking, "There's nothing that can be done anyway, so why bother? Better not to know." The message for you? Probe for symptoms, and encourage—if not take—your mom and dad to get regular checkups that screen for cancer. You also can reassure them that plenty of cancers can be stopped dead in their tracks—if you act in time. They also need to know that the therapies used today to treat cancer are far more advanced than the horror stories they might have heard or saw when they were younger. I recall how shocked I was when a colleague of mine came to work in the afternoon following his morning of chemotherapy. I, too, was back in the dark ages remembering how deathly ill my grandfather was after his chemotherapy. Your parents need to know how much times have changed!

Geri-Fact

Before I'm accused of presenting too rosy a picture, check out these statistics from the American Cancer Society:

- Cancer is the second leading cause of death in this country, exceeded only by heart disease.

- Every day, 1,500 people die of cancer. Every year, a million new cases of cancer are diagnosed.

- In the last 10 years, 5 million people lost their lives to cancer.

- Among the elderly, the top four cancers are lung, breast, prostate, and colon.

What Is Cancer?

Cancer is basically cells gone haywire. We have zillions of cells that grow and reproduce everyday. Cells get their orders on how to reproduce through the cell's DNA—kind of like a company's CEO. If cancer-causing substances like tobacco, alcohol, or some other toxins get to the CEO, his or her orders get hijacked. The message is mutilated and the cells that get this errant message start reproducing themselves. They aren't very popular with their co-workers (normal cells), so they take the hint and break away. They happily keep reproducing their mutated selves, and before you know it they've created their own spin-off company, what we call a tumor. Some of these tumors are satisfied just hanging out with themselves so they stay benign and harmless. But there are others that are very ambitious and they want to penetrate the market everywhere they can. These are the malignant guys. Their goal is to tear down their competition—their normal-cell neighbors—and take over your whole body. And that's a deadly scenario.

The Danger Signs

For years, the American Cancer Society has been warning us about the danger signs of cancer. Their message worked for me—I knew that a change in a mole was a sign and acted on it. Just to remind you, here's the list you and your parents need to keep in mind.

The Danger Signs of Cancer
(from the American Cancer Society)

- A sore that won't heal
- Obvious changes in a mole or wart
- Blood in the urine or persistent difficulty in urinating or having bowel movements
- Unusual and persistent constipation or a change in the usual frequency of bowel movements
- Persistent indigestion or stomach discomfort
- A sore throat and difficulty in swallowing
- Unusual bleeding or discharge anywhere in the body
- A nagging cough, hoarseness, difficulty in breathing, and coughing up blood in the sputum
- Pain that is persistent and without apparent cause
- A thickening or lump in the breast, vulva, neck, head, or other part of the body

Geri-Fact

At the time of diagnosis, you'll learn that the cancer is in one of four stages. Stage I is the most curable and Stage IV the least. These stages are used to grade the tumor itself (how large it is, whether it's affecting surrounding tissue, whether and to what extent the lymph nodes are involved, and how much the cancer has spread (metastasized).

If Mom or Dad complains of any of these symptoms, make sure he or she sees a primary physician. If you can't be with your parent during the appointment, most doctors will talk to you during or following the office visit. It's a good way to check on how your parent is doing and to make sure your parent didn't forget to bring up troublesome symptoms that he or she might think are just due to old age. Let your parent know you'll be calling. My Dad appreciates my sister getting on the phone because she's a nurse and can explain procedures to him, and she won't let him go through anything that isn't necessary.

Getting the Diagnosis

Whenever your parents are getting results of diagnostic tests, especially those to rule in or rule out cancer, you need to be there. If not physically, then by way of a conference call with the physician.

When people hear they have cancer—and I've been there—they find it pretty hard to soak in everything they're being told. It's like a stuck record—they can't get past the word "cancer." A cancer diagnosis will become a family affair, so you must be part of it early on.

Here are some questions you should ask the doctor:

- What's the medical name for this cancer? How do you spell it?
- How was the diagnosis made? Based on what tests?
- What stage is this cancer? Could you please explain the stages?
- Has the cancer spread (metastasized)? Where has it spread? Where did it originate—in other words, what is the primary site of the cancer?
- Can this cancer be cured?
- What treatments do you recommend?
- What's the goal of the treatment? Will it cure the cancer, stop it from spreading, reverse its effects, or simply make life more comfortable while it continues to spread?
- What are the side effects of the treatment? How will it affect other conditions that my parent has?
- What's the outlook (prognosis) for my parent?
- Could your office staff tell me if this treatment is covered under Medicare and my parent's Medi-gap policy?

Getting Treatment

No one is too old to receive some form of cancer treatment. Options range from managing pain and buying quality time to beating the cancer. Get involved in finding out about the wealth and range of treatment options for your parent's type of cancer. Work with your parent's doctor and do some homework on your own, too. Split the work up among your siblings. Have one person check out local support groups and treatment centers. Somebody else can surf the Net.

I've searched the Net for you and identified two excellent picks. The first place to call is the Information Service offered by the National Cancer Institute (NCI). They'll tell you about the nearest NCI designated cancer center that can treat your parent's type of cancer. By meeting the Institute's standards, these centers are up on the latest forms of treatment for specific cancers. The Institute will locate a center that's less than a day's drive away.

The NCI will also provide you with excellent information about your parent's cancer, including methods of diagnosis, staging, and treatment. They'll also tell you if a clinical trial is available to your parent.

Medicare is launching a new initiative to encourage more older folks to participate in clinical trials. Only 1 percent of the elderly participate in clinical trials, yet they are the ones who bear the brunt of the majority of the diseases in this country. Their participation is key to making future advances in medicine. If traditional treatment isn't working for your mom or dad, perhaps a clinical trial would be beneficial. There are some downsides. If the trial involves a control group that gets a "dummy" treatment known as a placebo, your parent could be assigned to the placebo group and not receive any treatment. Ask the physician to clearly explain to you the pluses and minuses of the trial. Medicare pays for all patient costs associated with a clinical trial and any complications that arise from it.

Never Too Old to Prevent Cancer

No one is too old to prevent cancer! You're never too old to stop smoking, take antioxidants such as Vitamin E, and eat a kick-cancer-butt diet of high fiber and low fat. Loads of research has been pouring in identifying the cancer culprits in the food we eat and the environment. Dietary habits are hard to break, no doubt about it, especially if your parents come from an ethnic background where fatty foods are celebrated (like my Irish roots of meat, potatoes, and lots of gravy). But as parents get older, they don't prepare big dinners every night. You could treat them to a catering service that delivers balanced meals on a weekly basis—your parents just pop the meals into the microwave or oven. Or if you're up to the task, do it yourself. You could also call Meals on Wheels at your local senior center, or offer to pay a neighbor who loves to cook.

Sage Source

There are two excellent organizations dedicated to cancer education and treatment. The first is the National Cancer Institute (1-800-4-CANCER or www.nci.nih.gov). Click on their Clinical Trials icon to find a clinical trial. The other is the American Cancer Society (1-800-ACS-2345 or www.cancer.org).

One of the best ways of staying ahead of cancer is to get regular checkups and cancer screenings. Your parents have absolutely no excuse for not being screened for breast, prostate, and colon cancer. These and other screenings are paid for by Medicare (see Chapter 21, "Got to Have Those M&Ms: Medicare and Medicaid").

More Options: Alternative Medicine

There are more options for your parent's treatment beyond the standard regimen of radiation, chemotherapy, and surgery offered by conventional, mainstream medicine. Complementary and alternative medicine (CAM) offers a wide array of health care practices, such as homeopathic, naturopathic, and Chinese medicine; biologically based therapies found in nature (herbs, foods, and vitamins); chiropractic or osteo-pathic manipulation; and energy therapies. Getting the mind and body to work effec-tively with its *own* natural healing process is the mantra of the alternative medicine crowd. Once you delve into this field, you'll learn about detoxifying the body so that the immune system can resume its job to fight the growth of cancer cells. Your Mom will need a good dose of personal responsibility and initiative if she's going to pursue this route. Make sure she shares what she's doing with her oncologist and primary physician. Conventional drugs (including chemotherapy) may not mix well with cer-tain herbs and vitamins, so keep everyone involved in your mother's care on the same page!

Please be aware that a good number of these methods have not gone through the rigors of Western scientific research, so you'll need to do your homework. This is not to say that what CAM has to offer is not effective. You just won't have the typical benchmarks to measure quality or safety. More major medical centers, however, are integrating CAM with conventional medicine. A good place to start your homework is the National Center for Complementary and Alternative Medicine's website at www.nccam.nih.gov, or call them toll free at 1-888-644-6226 for their Fact Sheets.

The Least You Need to Know

- Sometimes symptoms of Alzheimer's are really a reaction to drugs. Before you assume anything, have a doctor (preferably a geriatrician) examine your parent.

- Parents in their late 80s have nearly a 50 percent chance of suffering from dementia.

- You might need to probe your parents for cancer symptoms. Too many in their generation feel that "What you don't know won't hurt you."

- Medicare covers cancer screening tests and all patient costs associated with clinical trials.

- If your parent is diagnosed with cancer, be part of their care. Go to doc-tor's appointments with them. If you can't be there, ask the doctor to call you when they've finished examining your parent.

Part 2

The World of Geriatric Health Care

Keeping up with the Joneses is a lot easier than keeping up with today's health care system. Every day you hear about mergers, IPOs, PPOs, HMOs (alphabet soup, anyone?), and managed care plans that are pulling the plug. And trying to help your parents at a distance makes it a double whammy.

But we're here to help. You'll learn how to manage the health care maze that your parent is caught up in, even if you live far away. We'll help you navigate a hospital stay, find good home health care, and give you a mini-course on being a patient advocate for your parents.

Your mom and dad are more at risk of having an adverse drug reaction than any other age group in this country. Learn how to stay on top of their prescriptions and keep them out of the hospital. And yes, there are ways to get prescriptions without paying an arm and a leg. We'll show you how.

Chapter 7

Managing the Health Care Maze—Even from a Distance

In This Chapter

- Organizing your parent's health care information
- Geriatric assessments and geriatricians
- Coming up with a family plan to care for your parents
- Long-distance caregiving tips
- Geriatric care managers to the rescue

The older you get, the more doctors you visit. Before you know it, your body turns into an employment agency for specialists: heart doctors, foot doctors, arthritis doctors, eye doctors, hearing doctors, cancer doctors, diabetes doctors, and a good old general doctor. Trust me, Mom isn't all that excited about all of the attention. If she has a good general practitioner who takes charge of all of the specialists, coordinates all of her care and the pills each of them prescribes, she's ahead of the game.

But far too many older people see each specialist in a world of their own … the doctor's world. As a result, Mom's body is treated in bits and pieces. For some parents this can be overwhelming and for most, this isn't the best way to receive treatment. All those systems in Mom's body work together in a very intricate way, and so should all the doctors treating her. But many times, they don't. And that's where you come in.

Getting Organized

Somehow "Things to Do" lists and scraps of paper with notes on them, elude me. They run off somewhere just like the socks in the dryer—at least one sock. So, I've learned that the best way to get control of these runaway notes is to contain them. You'll find that if you get involved in your parent's medical care, the notes will pile up quickly. And so will the forms, insurance papers, and information on each condition affecting your parents. So get a handle on this early and buy an expandable file that can hold about 10 folders. Here's how I'd go about organizing them:

- Insurance papers: copies of contacts, ID numbers.
- Each physician: Place the name and phone number of each doctor on the outside of a folder. Keep notes of your conversations and any material given by physician.
- Medications list and any material about the medications such as copies of drug package inserts and any materials the pharmacist gave with the medication.
- Copies of your parents' living wills and their health care power of attorney.
- Background material on each condition (a diabetic folder, high blood pressure, and so on).
- Master contact list: Make one master list that you can work from that includes names and phone numbers of your parents' physicians, home health care workers, insurance companies, pharmacist, hospital social worker, area agency on aging, neighbors, and any community agency or group (home-delivered meals, for example) that interacts your parents. List Medicare, Social Security, and insurance ID numbers.
- Copies of Social Security, Medicare, and Medicaid cards and any insurance cards that your parent has to present at doctors' offices.
- Home health care and community services names and phone numbers and brochures describing their services.
- Hospital information: Pick up a copy of the directory of the hospital your parents use and keep it in the folder.

By gathering the information for each folder, you'll be identifying the kinds of things you need to know to help organize your parents' care. As you'll learn in Chapter 8, "Pills and Your Parents," one of the leading causes of hospitalizations among the elderly is adverse drug reactions. It's really important for you to know all of the pills your mom and dad are taking. Read and maintain the drug package inserts that spell out possible problems with the drugs. Make sure all of your parents' doctors know what they're taking, including over-the-counter drugs. Whenever a prescribed drug has caused problems, note that in the drug folder. But enough said here, the next chapter will fill you in on the medications scene.

Geriatric Assessments—Getting the Lay of the Land

One way to deal with the maze of health care is to control it from the start. Rather than having Mom bounce around from one specialist to the next, it's best to get a full read of just what ails her from someone who really understands the intricacies of her body—a *geriatrician*. If your mom is in an HMO (managed care plan), her primary physician will need to make the referral. If, not, you can request her family doctor make a referral, or you can find a geriatrician on your own.

Medical centers that conduct full-scale *geriatric* assessments are your best bet to get your mom or dad a complete workup. A full assessment can take from three hours to two days of testing. If your parent's health is beginning to decline, if he or she has three or more chronic conditions that require a good degree of maintenance, or if your parent is taking more than five maintenance medications and you're not sure what's going on, it's a good idea to get a geriatric assessment.

Unlike most physical exams, a geriatric assessment assesses your parent's physical functioning. The physician will evaluate his or her range of motion, ability to walk, reach, bend, maintain balance, and manage steps, and his or her degree of difficulty getting in and out of a chair.

Geri-Fact

Geriatrics (derived from the Greek *geras*, meaning "old age") is the medical science of the physical and mental processes of aging. A **geriatrician** is a medical doctor certified in geriatrics. This is different from a gerontologist, which is an individual who has studied the field of aging from a social science perspective. Gerontologists are not physicians.

An interdisciplinary team will get involved in the evaluation. For example, nutritionists will look at your parent's dietary needs and habits, and an occupational therapist will evaluate how your parent functions in the activities of daily living. Pharmacists will look over all of the pills Mom or Dad takes to determine if the combination of pills, dosages, and duration are working well together. Other specialists will be brought in to evaluate your parent's unique needs, especially if something is picked up during the assessment.

Another major component of the geriatric assessment is an evaluation of your parent's cognitive functioning (thinking ability). The doctor will ask Mom or Dad a variety of abstract questions and will test for memory (a Mini-Mental Status Exam). The doctor will test for any signs of dementia or confusion (see Chapter 6, "Alzheimer's Disease and Cancer," for more on dementia). Social workers and psychiatrists will also assess your mom and dad's mental health to rule out depression or other mental disorders.

Silver Lining

Before your parent goes for the assessment, think about how your parent functions during the day. Consider areas of difficulty, any symptoms he or she is experiencing, your parent's chronic conditions and treatment used for each (include physician names), family history of physical and mental disease, a list of all drugs your parent takes, allergies, sleeping patterns, alcohol and tobacco use, past injuries, and hospitalizations. If Mom or Dad is experiencing confusion, check The Top Ten Warning Signs of Alzheimer's Disease list in Chapter 6 and mention your parent's symptoms to the assessment team.

At the foundation of all this study will be a series of tests (EKGs, blood work, scans, neurological tests) to determine if there are any physiological reasons for the symptoms or conditions that your parent reports. Once all the testing, interviewing, and exams are completed, the team meets to discuss what they've learned about your parent. They then present their findings and come up with a care plan to meet your parent's needs that were identified through the assessment. Most geriatric centers also offer treatment and can become the manager of your parent's care. Others provide the results of the geriatric assessment to your parent's primary physician to assist him or her in overseeing your parent's care.

Sage Source

To find a geriatric assessment center near your parent, call your local hospitals. Most university-based hospitals have a geriatric specialty and perform such assessments. You can also call the American Geriatrics Society at 212-308-1414, or visit their Web site at www.americangeriatrics. org. They can send you a list of physicians certified in geriatrics or e-mail information to you.

Geriatricians

If you're not able to find a geriatric center, you may be able to track down physicians who are in private practice or practice in a group that specializes in geriatrics. Some family practice doctors and internists have received certification in geriatrics by taking special courses and passing an exam. Ask the physician if he or she has a fellowship or received certification in geriatrics. The benefit offered by a physician who has specialized in geriatrics is the ability to "piece things together." The physician understands the physiological changes of aging, and knows what's normal and what's not. The physician has a better appreciation of how medications interact with your mom or dad's physiological changes. This is important because many drugs have not been tested on elderly people.

Coming Up with a Family Plan

Once you have a complete picture of your parent's physical and mental needs, it's time for the family to come together and determine how best to meet those needs.

If your parent is competent, include Mom or Dad in the discussion. As you'll see through various sections of this book, there are plenty of options depending upon your parent's level of dependency.

Caring for Mom and Dad should be a family affair where everybody pitches in. Even those who live far away can assist by making phone calls, researching information on the Internet, or tracking down and ordering assistive devices to make life easier. Another can keep track of all the paperwork (such as insurance papers) or assist with contacting physicians, homemakers, or home health services. Once you've decided who does what, put it in writing and share it with each other.

As you work through the health care maze, you'll find you'll need to become an advocate for your parents. Far too many of their generation think that the doctor's always right or they simply don't know what to ask. Decide among you who would make the best spokesperson to negotiate the "system." It gets too confusing if you and your siblings are all calling the doctor. If you need to, make use of three-way calling or even a conference call when talking with a physician. And as families become more adept with e-mail, it makes for a very good way to keep the communication channels open. Part 4, "Caregiving: Coming to Live with You," offers more tips on working together when one of you cares for a parent at home.

Sage Source

The American Board of Internal Medicine can send you a list of all the internists in your state who have received certification in geriatrics. They take only written requests submitted through the mail or by fax, at 215-446-3590. Mail requests to The American Board of Internal Medicine, 510 Walnut Street, Suite 1700, Philadelphia, PA 19106. You can also call your local hospital or nursing home for a referral.

Senior Alert

Stay focused on Mom or Dad's needs and wants. Let go of unsettled arguments with Mom or Dad. Stick to a things-to-do list that focuses on the tasks to help Mom and Dad.

Long-Distance Caregiving

It's pretty rare these days for immediate family members to be living in one place. When you add on the remarriages of parents *and* adult children, it gets even more complicated. If your parents live far away, making sure that they are being taken care of presents its own set of problems. But with thoughtful planning and smart advance work, you can be very effective at being the good son or daughter they deserve.

Advance Work

Advance teams for political campaigns can make or break an event—and a candidate. It's their job to scope out the town, know the hot-button issues in that community, get everybody's name right, know who to invite, and brief the candidate. You'll need to do somewhat of the same. Think of it as your parents' campaign to make it on their own. They're the candidates and you're the advance team. Here's what you do:

- **Get to know the neighbors.** Identify one or two neighbors whom you trust who will look in on your parent on a regular basis. Exchange phone numbers so that you can call them if you become concerned about your mom or dad, and they can call you. If you and your parent are comfortable with the arrangement, give them a set a keys. Make sure the neighbor's phone number is programmed on your parent's phone, so he or she is just a button away from fast access.

- **Get to know the mail carrier.** The mail carrier is in a position to notice if Mom or Dad has stopped picking up the mail. Many post offices and utility companies have elder-watch programs that will alert the area agency on aging to contact family members if they suspect a problem. Contact the area agency on aging to sign your parent up for such a program.

- **Get to know the bankers.** Maybe it's a good thing, after all, that our parents' generation still likes the good old human touch of a bank teller and bank manager. An ATM machine sure won't give you a call that Mom or Dad has been asking to take out large sums of money. Or that a stranger accompanied them when he opened his safety deposit box. Introduce yourself to the banking staff and give them your phone number to call you if they think something is amiss.

- **Get to know your parent's best friends.** My husband and I both have mothers who live alone in Phoenix. We're in Philadelphia. We have a list of friends for each of our Mom's and when we go to visit, we make it a point to keep up with their friends. We've each had occasions to call those friends when our moms needed help until we could get there. Our moms are both in pretty good health, active, and independent. Yet, when they have the flu or a medical problem hits, it's good to call on some friends who will get groceries, fix some chicken soup, and look in on them. They can also become your eyes and ears, alerting you to changes and concerns that you won't pick up in a phone call or even during a short visit. They'll be more inclined to open up to you if you've developed a relationship with them, too. So, include them on a visit and bring a plant or flowers to show your appreciation.

- **Get to know the community services.**
Call the local United Way to get a directory of community services in your parent's area. Call the local senior center to find out what services are available for your parent. And of course, get the phone number of the area agency on aging. Be sure to save all of their background material and place it in your folder (see "Getting Organized" earlier in this chapter). Get to know the eligibility criteria prior to actually needing the service. That way you won't lose precious time or be "in the dark" as to what is available to your parent when the need hits.

Silver Lining

If your parent is on a limited income or frets over the costs of long-distance bills, consider getting an 800 number so Mom or Dad will feel free to call you.

- **Get to know the home health services network.** You'll need to get to know the home health services network available to your parent, so that when Mom or Dad need it you can spring into action. If your parent is using home health care, be sure to call every day to get a report on how he or she is doing. See Chapter 10, "Home Health Care," for specifics.

- **Bring home the phone book!** A good advance team has everybody's phone numbers. So next time you're visiting, bring back an extra copy of your parents' local phone book. The Yellow Pages are especially helpful. If you're online, there are a number of Web sites that offer phone book services, such as www.yellowpages.com.

- **Set up a chore services network.** If your parents need help mowing the lawn, shoveling snow, walking the dog, or keeping up with minor house repairs, see if there is a neighbor or local college student who can be paid to help out. If you need to go a more formal route, contact the area agency on aging to see if they can identify someone for you. Chapter 12, "Living in the Community: Services and Transportation," is chock full of resources to help your parents remain at home.

Making Your Visit Count

It seems like there are never enough hours in the day, especially when you visit family and try to sneak in visiting old friends. You'll need to make the most of your visit and use your sensors to pick up potential trouble. Sometimes it's very obvious that

Mom has become confused, lost weight, appears depressed, or is having difficulty getting around. But many times, the changes are subtle and you have to be especially adept at picking up the clues. These questions can help you do your own mini-assessment:

- Is mail left unopened or are newspapers piled up?
- Are the bills being paid?
- Is Mom or Dad ordering an excessive amount of things from catalogs, from insurance companies, or from television infomercials?
- If Mom or Dad has been active, determine whether or not his or her activity level has remained the same. When was the last time your parent visited friends? Went out?
- What's in the refrigerator? Spoiled food? Too little food?
- How much does Mom repeat herself? Does she question you after you've just explained something a short while before? Does she give you the impression that she's not retaining what you say?
- If you take a trip to the mall or a restaurant, notice if Dad's having any difficulty calculating discounts or tips, writing a check, or figuring out change, or hands over a $10 bill thinking it's a $1 bill.

Silver Lining

If you handle your parents' finances, send them large, stamped, self-addressed envelopes so that they can just drop in bills and send them on to you. Better yet, get your parents on an automatic bill paying system and have their Social Security, pension, and other income checks electronically deposited.

Senior Alert

If you're visiting a sibling who takes care of your parent, be sure to schedule time so that he or she can take a break from the caregiving.

Arrange physician visits around your trips. Let the doctor's office know that you'll be coming in from out of town. Many doctors will squeeze you in if they know you are traveling from out of town to be there. Even if this is a routine office visit, it's more helpful if you're there to ask questions and bring up points that your mom or dad might forget. Be sure to leave your phone number with the doctor so that he or she can call you to alert you to any changes in your parent's condition.

Cyber Seniors: Staying in Touch via Computer

Before you fall into old stereotypes about teaching old dogs new tricks, you should know that the elderly are the fastest-growing group on the Internet. (Just check out AOL's recent ads with two older ladies talking about their e-mail with their grandkids!) Get Mom and Dad a computer or WebTV (in which they can use their TV to go online for a monthly fee).

You or one of your kids could provide the training to get your parents up and running. Or get your parent to sign up for a class at the local community college or senior center. Many older folks find using the Web very exciting and informative, especially as a source of information on their health conditions. The American Association of Retired Persons (AARP) Web site at www.aarp.org is a terrific resource. Another benefit of having a computer or WebTV is using e-mail, which is an excellent way for your parents to stay in touch with the whole family, especially Internet-savvy grandkids. You can even get them a small video cam (you'll need to buy one, too) so that they can see you every day.

Geriatric Care Managers

Meet the new kid on the block in geriatrics. Realizing the need to coordinate the multiple layers of care that older people require, social workers, counselors, and nurses have created a new field of geriatrics: care management. Besides meeting the needs of parents, they also address the needs of baby boomers who are caught up in long-distance care giving. Here's what geriatric care managers can do:

- Conduct an assessment of your parent to identify the kinds of care your parent needs.

- Determine eligibility for various services, contact the services, and process papers.

- Interview, arrange, and monitor home care workers and other services provided in the home to your parent.

- Provide referrals to other geriatric specialists and/or set up an appointment for a geriatric assessment.

- Arrange for transportation to and from appointments and services.

- Provide crisis intervention counseling.

- Oversee moving your parent from home to an assisted living residence, nursing home, or retirement community.

- Analyze financial, legal, or medical information and interpret it for family members so that they understand their options.

- Become a liaison between your parent and yourself by monitoring your parent's condition through home visits and reporting back to you.

- Research quality of care inspection reports of nursing homes, personal care homes, and community care retirement communities and provide you with the results.

What Do Geriatric Care Managers Charge?

At the present time, insurance companies do not pick up the costs of geriatric care management. You'll have to pay for this on your own. Despite the cost, however, the manager can save you money by knowing of services your parent may qualify for, by being very knowledgeable of Medicare and Medicaid, and by having access to community services. The manager can also save you the costs of travel and lost time searching for care.

Fees can range from $50 to $150 per hour depending upon the care manager's credentials and experience. Some charge by the hour while others charge set fees for a package of services. The initial assessment may cost from $150 to $350 and then, based upon your parent's needs, you and the care manager decide upon a monthly fee.

Questions to Ask a Potential Care Manager

When you interview a geriatric care manager, here are some questions you'll want to ask:

- What services do you provide?
- What are your credentials? Are you licensed in your profession?
- How long have you been providing care management services? How long have you been practicing in this community?
- Do you have any affiliations and memberships in community organizations?
- Are you available for emergencies? Who do you have on backup if you aren't available?
- What can I expect to learn from your initial assessment?
- How do you know that the services you recommend or make referrals to meet high quality standards?
- How do you communicate information to me about my parent?

Senior Alert

Individuals who present themselves as geriatric care managers are not regulated by any governmental or professional body, because the profession is still new. If a care manager is a social worker or nurse, he or she should have a state license in the respective profession. Ask if the person is licensed and belongs to any professional associations, and be sure to get references.

Sage Source

Living Strategies is a new eldercare solutions company that will track down a geriatric care manager for you and oversee his or her work. Visit them at www.livingstrategies.com. For a list of geriatric care managers in your area, contact The National Association of Professional Geriatric Care Managers at 520-881-8008 or www.caremanager.org. You can also check the Yellow Pages under Social Workers, or your local area agency on aging.

- How often will you have face-to-face contact with my parent?
- How many cases do you handle at one time?
- What are your fees? Can you provide me with references?

Care management is often provided free or at a minimal cost for low-income individuals by area agencies on aging, senior centers, and other community service organizations. Call your local area agency on aging to find out if your parent qualifies.

The Least You Need to Know

- A geriatric assessment is an excellent way for an interdisciplinary team to get a comprehensive view of exactly what's going on with your parent's physical and mental health.

- Geriatricians are physicians who specialize in the medical and health care of the elderly.

- Everyone in the family can play a role in caring for your parents, even if they live out of town. Create a things-to-do list and share the tasks among family members.

- Long-distance caregiving has its challenges, but with smart advance work and creative solutions, you can be very effective in helping your mom and dad.

- Geriatric care managers can arrange for, coordinate, and monitor your parent's care. They are especially helpful if you live out of town.

Pills and Your Parents

The right pill in the right amount for the right reason can do wonders for your parents. That little tiny capsule can keep them alive, keep them out of a nursing home, help them get to sleep or make them feel like a million dollars. Or it can land them smack-dab into the emergency room—or even the grave.

With the average older adult getting 18 prescriptions filled every year and spending thousands of dollars out of their own pockets—staying on top of drug safety and costs can be a full-time job. It's my hope that by reading this chapter, you'll save time, money, and a trip to the hospital.

Seniors on Drugs

No, I'm not talking about seniors in high school or college. America's "other drug problem" is among seniors 65 years-plus. These seniors are swallowing one-third of all the prescriptions out there yet they make up only 13 percent of the population. And this doesn't include the over-the-counter (OTC) drugs that the senior crowd takes like aspirin, cold medicines, antacids, vitamins, and laxatives. On that front, they buy 40 percent of all the OTC drugs in the country.

Geri-Fact

A recent study in the *Journal of the American Medical Association* reported that drug reactions kill an estimated 100,000 people a year in U.S. hospitals. The researchers also claim that another 2.1 million are injured by adverse reactions. The elderly are especially vulnerable because of the number of drugs they take.

Senior Alert

One of the more common side effects of multiple medications is dizziness and confusion. Before anyone decides Dad now has Alzheimer's, make sure his physician rules out medications as a factor. Some doctors put their patients on a "drug holiday" slowly taking them off all drugs to determine exactly what's going on.

Drugs That Don't Get Along

The most dangerous problem that older adults face when taking drugs is how multiple drugs interact with each other. One quarter of the elderly take at least three drugs a day. The older they are, the more drugs they take. The more drugs they take, the greater the risk in having the combination of drugs kick off a significant health problem.

Chances are your mom and dad have more than one chronic condition, so they get to meet a number of specialists. As they visit one doctor after the next, they might walk away from each visit with a prescription in hand. If they forgot to tell either doctor about what they're taking, they've placed themselves in danger of an adverse drug reaction. Besides taking drugs that may negatively interact with each other, your parents might also be taking the same drug twice—and not know it.

One doctor might give a drug in the *generic* name and another in the *brand name*. Our parents might think that they are taking two separate drugs because the names are very different and the pills don't look alike. If the doctors are unaware of what Mom or Dad is taking, or your pharmacist doesn't pick up the double whammy, your parents could be in for some serious trouble.

Not all drugs or combinations of drugs are bad. For instance, a physician might prescribe an anti-ulcer medication with an anti-inflammatory medication. The doctor is doing this because the anti-inflammatory drug can cause severe irritation to the lining of the stomach. So as a precautionary measure, he or she will prescribe the anti-ulcer drug.

Geri-Fact

A **generic** drug is labeled by its chemical name, while a **brand name** drug carries a name given by its manufacturer. For example, the brand name of the sleeping medication Restoril has a generic equivalent known as temazepam. Generics are spinoffs of brand name drugs, but they must have the same active ingredients, strength, and dosage form as brand name drugs. They must also be the same chemically and have the same medical effect. Generics cost much less than the brand name drug, sometimes half the price.

Not Following Directions

Medication mishaps don't always come from seeing too many doctors and a lack of communication. Older pill takers have a reputation for not following directions. Studies show that three out of four older adults don't take their medications properly. A quarter of all nursing home admissions are linked to an inability to correctly take medications. They are labeled in the medical community as being "noncompliant." It's not like they mean to be this way. If Dad has arthritis and finds it a pain to open the pill bottle, is forgetful, or has poor eyesight and can't read the small print, he'll have problems keeping up with his drug regimen. When it comes to taking three or four pills a day—each one at a different time and a different number of times throughout the day—it's no wonder. Always check with your parent's doctor if you have any questions or concerns about their medications.

Over-the-Counter Drugs

To add to the pharmaceutical pot, your parents are also buying over-the-counter drugs that can negatively interact with prescribed drugs. All too often, your parents won't think of telling the doctor that they're taking aspirin, antacids, cold medicines, and laxatives. If Dad is taking a blood-thinning medication and aspirins, he's going overboard on the thinners and can risk hemorrhaging. Those Tums for Mom's calcium can cause real havoc with her medicine for Parkinson's disease. Though most of these OTC drugs are safe, they are not risk free. More than 600 of these drugs contain ingredients and dosages that 20 years ago you couldn't even buy *without* a doctor's prescription. Just because Mom and Dad can buy pills over the counter, doesn't mean they're not drugs.

Different Bodies, Different Doses

Silver Lining

Soon you'll see clearly marked and understandable labels on all over-the-counter drugs. Thanks to the Food and Drug Administration (FDA), drug companies must use simple language to explain the risks of the drug, print the risks in large type, and present the information in a standardized, easy-to-follow format on the outside of the package. It will be similar to the food labels we now have on all food products. So read the labels!

The aging body has something to say about all this pill popping. That vintage body can't take the same dosage as a young body. The kidney and liver—big players in processing drugs in the body—slow down with age. Less muscle tissue and more fat tissue in the geriatric body means that drug absorption rates get skewed. How long the drug stays in the body, how fast it gets through the system, and how quickly it's eliminated all play a part in how well Mom or Dad tolerates a drug. Be aware that most drugs have been tested on young people (although this practice is beginning to change). As a result, doctors and drug companies have to guesstimate what's an appropriate dose for older people. Dad's physician may start his dosage low and slowly work up to an amount that meets your Dad's unique needs. It's a smart move.

Working with Doctors

Taking medications must be a cooperative effort between your parents and their doctors. Passively taking pills as they go from one doctor to another isn't smart or safe. Mom and Dad have to ask questions and give information. They should do this at every visit.

When a physician gives your parents new medication, here's what they should be *asking*:

- What is the name of the medication (brand name *and* generic name)?
- What is the medication supposed to do?
- Why are you recommending that I take this?
- How often should I take the drug?
- How long should I take the drug?
- When should I take it? (Whenever I need to? Before, during, or after meals? At bedtime?)

- Should I avoid certain foods or alcohol when taking this drug? Should I stay out of the sun?

- Should this medicine be refrigerated?

- If I forget to take it, what should I do?

- What side effects might I expect? Under what circumstances should I call you?

- Is there any written material on this drug?

- Is there something else I could try first, such as a change in diet, exercise, or therapy?

- How much does this drug cost? (Let the doctor know if you cannot afford it. Ask if there is a generic substitute, which costs less.)

And here's what your parents should be *telling* their physician:

- The name of all prescription drugs they are taking, including how long and how frequently they're taken.

- Any over-the-counter drugs they're taking, including vitamins.

- All allergies to medications and food.

- Any serious side effect they've had to a particular medication.

- If Mom or Dad has stopped taking a medication, your parent can't keep it a secret. The doctor needs to know since some medications work in combination with other drugs.

- Any concern about not being able to afford the medication.

If your parents take quite a few medications, make a copy of the following Pill Tracking Chart and have your parents or you bring it to every physician visit. The doc will really appreciate it because it will save time and provide the information he or she needs to assess what's going on.

Working with Pharmacists

Most pharmacists are eager to give you information, if you just ask. You and your parents will find it helpful to ask the pharmacist the same list of questions that you asked the doctor. Hearing it twice and double-checking doesn't hurt. The pharmacist is also a great resource to ask about over-the-counter drugs. Many pharmacies have additional consumer-friendly information on the drugs that they dispense, so ask for a copy. Thanks to the computer age, almost all pharmacies keep a profile on what drugs you

Sage Source

Want to know the skinny on the drugs you or your parents take? Check out the National Library of Medicine's Web site at www. nlm.nih.gov/medlineplus. It offers a guide to 9,000 prescription and over-the-counter medications.

take and all of your allergies. When you're given a new medication be sure to ask the pharmacist to run a scan on your profile to make sure that you won't have a problem with the new drug. The pharmacist is also the most up-to-date person on whether or not there is a generic available for the drug you've been prescribed. (You usually don't have to check with your doctor to substitute a generic.)

Pill Tracking Chart

Patient Name: _____

Date of Birth: _____

Allergies: _____

_____

Name of Prescription Drug	How Many Pills a Day?	What Time of Day
_____	_____	_____
_____	_____	_____
_____	_____	_____
_____	_____	_____
_____	_____	_____
_____	_____	_____

Name of Over-the-Counter Drug	How Many Pills a Day?	What Time of Day
_____	_____	_____
_____	_____	_____
_____	_____	_____
_____	_____	_____
_____	_____	_____

"I'd Rather Fight Than Switch"

Pharmacy benefit managers (PBMs) are companies hired by insurance companies, employers, and HMOs to oversee their drug benefit plans. PBMs make sure that insured individuals don't use too many or too expensive drugs. Drug companies that give price breaks or rebates get on a list, called a formulary, with the PBMs. In return, the PBMs steer pharmacists toward those drugs on which the PBMs received a better price. It's possible a PBM will tell the pharmacist to switch your prescription to the drug on its formulary.

Senior Alert

If your parent's insurance company or Medicare managed care plan has asked the pharmacist to switch the drug to something different (other than a generic) from what the physician prescribed, tell the pharmacist you want to know! Ask him or her to explain the difference between the two drugs. If your parent doesn't adjust well to the drug the insurance plan says he or she must take, let the doctor know. Ask the doctor to call the insurance plan to get your parent back on his or her proper medication.

But here's the problem: Many of these PBMs have financial relationships with drug companies and, in fact, a significant number are *owned* by drug companies. The FDA is now investigating conflict of interest issues and whether these switches are causing adverse reactions for patients. Physicians and elderly advocates across the country want a full investigation. According to studies conducted by the American Medical Association, millions of Americans are at risk because of this practice and already have been hurt by adverse drug reactions. If your parent has been doing well on a medication and all of a sudden he or she is told to switch, look into it. If your parent would rather fight than switch, let the physician know what's going on and file an appeal with your insurance carrier.

Silver Lining

Your mom or dad may be eligible to participate in a clinical trial where he or she will receive free medications and medical care. This is very helpful if your parent has a special condition for which current treatment practices aren't effective. These clinical trials are overseen by the FDA and are conducted by medical groups and universities throughout the country. To find a clinical trial that might help your parent, visit a National Institutes of Health Web site at www.clinicaltrials.gov that tracks trials down for you by condition and location. Be aware, though, that your parent might be chosen to get the "dummy" pill known as the placebo.

Tips on Taking Meds

Swallowing a pill seems simple enough. But, as in most things, there's more to it than meets the eye. Here are some tips your parents need to keep in mind:

- Don't share your medications with your spouse or friends.
- Take the full dosage for the time prescribed. Don't quit as soon as you feel better.
- Don't take fewer medications per day to stretch out the prescription.
- If you're not feeling better or are reacting poorly to the drug, call your physician.
- If you're taking multiple drugs, set up a system to keep track of what you are taking and when. Check them off as you go.
- Discard expired medications. It's too easy to confuse old medicine bottles with new ones.

Sage Source

The National Library of Medicine's www.nlm.nih.gov/medlineplus is a great Web site for up-to-date consumer information on medications, over-the-counter drugs, and new discoveries. It also offers terrific links and related information.

- If the prescription bottle is too hard to open or too small, ask your pharmacist to dispense it in a bigger bottle with large print and an easy-to-open cap.
- Ask your pharmacist about devices that can help you keep track of your medicines. (The pharmacist calls them compliance aids.) To name a few, there are check-off calendars, containers for daily doses, and bottle caps that beep when it's time to take a dose.
- Here's a shocker: Don't store your prescriptions in the medicine cabinet! Turns out, the bathroom is too warm and humid. Pills should be stored in cool and dry places.

Buying Medications on the Internet

Cyber pills. You knew it had to come. Instead of getting your pills at the friendly corner drugstore, you're a click away to online buying. There are certainly some advantages to getting your meds online:

- Easy access for homebound elderly
- Easy comparative shopping for the best price

- Access to a great variety of products
- Ability to consult with a pharmacist and order products in the privacy of your own home

The FDA, however, warns that there are a growing number of rogue sites that are downright dangerous. They'll send you pills without a prescription, which is *never* a good idea. Or they'll have you fill out a questionnaire, then tell you that a doctor has looked over your symptoms and recommends the following medication—when no such doctor ever looked it over!

In a famous national case, a man ordered Viagra online. He also had a history of chest pains and a family history of heart disease. All he did was fill out an online questionnaire. He died of a heart attack as soon as he started taking the drug. Though there is no direct proof that the man's death was linked to the drug, FDA officials contend that a traditional doctor-patient relationship with a good physical may have prevented the death. In the meantime, Congress is scrambling to keep up with online drug buying and come up with legislation to regulate it for the public's safety, just as they regulate pharmacies.

So, what if you want this convenience and still be assured it's safe? Here's some safe Internet buying tips from the FDA:

- Check with the National Association of Boards of Pharmacy to make sure that the site is a licensed pharmacy in good standing. Visit the Web site at www.nabp.net/vipps, or call 847-698-6227.
- Stay clear of sites that offer to prescribe a prescription for a drug the first time without a physical exam.
- Don't buy from sites that sell prescription drugs without a prescription or that sell drugs not approved by the FDA.
- Beware of sites that advertise a new cure for a serious disorder or a quick cure-all for lots of ailments. It's cyber snake oil!
- Don't do business with sites that don't provide you access to a registered pharmacist.
- For any first-time drug—always go through your physician first.

In general, legitimate online pharmacies will ask you to open an account with them, and then submit credit and insurance information. They'll ask you to submit a valid prescription which your doctor can call in, fax, or mail. The online pharmacy can ship it to you, or you can pick it up at a local drugstore. Most sites have an online registered pharmacist to whom you can e-mail questions or can reach at a toll-free number.

Saving Money on Prescriptions

It certainly isn't a news flash that prescriptions these days cost an arm and a leg. Medicare doesn't pick up the tab on pills (unless you're in the hospital), insurance is expensive, and prices continue to skyrocket. A recent study by the nonprofit consumer advocacy group Families USA confirmed that the prices of drugs most frequently used by older Americans rose 30 percent on average over the last six years. It's not uncommon for people to shell out $2,000 to $3,000 a year on prescription drugs.

It's no wonder so many older folks are up in arms over drug prices. My mother, in order to get pain medicine for my dying stepfather, had to use her charge card to buy 10 pills for a staggering $800. He died four days later. At least she had the credit to cover the costs. As Secretary of Aging, I met hundreds of older people who had to walk away from the pharmacy because they simply couldn't afford to pay. Others paid their utility bills late, shut off the air-conditioning, or went without food in order to buy the medications. Hopefully, you're not in that situation but with no end in sight of rising drug prices, it's to your advantage to become a smart consumer. Check out my Prescription for Saving on Medications:

Silver Lining

Help out the Feds! If you think you've come across an illegal pharmacy Web site, let the FDA know by e-mailing them at webcomplaints@ora.fda.gov.

- Ask if there is a generic equivalent of the drug being prescribed. Generics are less expensive than the brand name drug, sometimes as little as half the price.

- If your parent is taking a new drug for the *first* time, ask for a trial size rather than a 30-day supply. That way if you have an adverse reaction to the drug, you won't be throwing away your money and the pills for a full 30-day supply. If the drug is working well, you'll need to ask your doctor for a refill to finish the prescription.

- Ask the doctor for drug samples. In most cases, the doctor will be able to get you started on a drug with free samples provided by the drug company.

- If your parent is taking a maintenance drug—a drug Mom or Dad has to take for a long time to maintain health—look into buying in quantity. A 90-day supply will be cheaper than a month's supply.

- Look into ordering maintenance drugs by mail or online. They are usually cheaper than they would be at a drug store because there is less overhead. If you're ordering online (see the previous section, "Buying Medications on the Internet"), make sure it's a credible group that has been approved by the National Association of Boards of Pharmacy. Visit www.nabp.net/vipps to see if they're okay.

- Shop around. Call pharmacies to find out their prices for various medications. You'd be surprised at the difference. Many will deliver for free, so you won't have to travel all over town to get the best buy. Also ask them if they offer senior citizen discounts.

- If your parent must take medications over the long term (for diabetes, blood pressure, Parkinson's, or cardiovascular problems, for example), look into an insurance plan. If the monthly premiums and deductibles are less than what they put out every month—go for it.

- Some states have prescription assistance programs for low and moderate income elderly. Call the local area agency on aging to find out how to qualify for any programs in your state or visit www.rxassist.org or www.benefitscheckup.org.

- Some drug companies offer free or reduced-price medications in certain cases. Visit www.phrma.org to see if the manufacturer of your parent's drug participates. Only your parent's physician can apply to the drug company on your parent's behalf. It doesn't hurt for you to do the homework and share the information with your parent's physician so he or she can apply on your parent's behalf.

- If your parent receives prescriptions in a nursing home from the facility's pharmacist be sure to scan the monthly bill. Many homes inflate the prices. Instead, you can choose to buy them on your own and have your parent's medications delivered to the nursing home.

The Least You Need to Know

- It's estimated that 100,000 people die from adverse drug reactions and millions of others are injured from them every year.

- When taking medications, it's crucial that your parents work closely with their doctor and pharmacist, to ask questions and offer information.

- If your parent has been doing well on a medication and then is suddenly told to switch, check with your parent's doctor right away.

- If your parent takes multiple drugs, set up a system to keep track of what Mom or Dad is taking and at what time. Always take the full dosage for the entire time prescribed.

- Buying medications online offers many benefits, but be alert to scams.

- There's plenty you can do to save money when buying medications.

A Trip to the Hospital

If I were a fortune teller studying your 80-year-old mom's palms, I might predict that a hospital stay is in her near future. Chances are I'd be right and you'd think I was pretty good.

But all I had to do was know that 50 percent of people over 80 will enter a hospital this year, and there's a one in four chance that anyone over 65 years will be admitted to a hospital. With these kinds of odds, it's a good idea for you to become very familiar with the ins and outs (literally) of hospitals.

Finding the Right Hospital

Hopefully, your parent's hospital stay allows for a bit of planning rather than an emergency admission. Your parent's primary physician and/or surgeon will usually recommend a hospital where they have admitting privileges, meaning that the doctor has been approved by the hospital to practice there. Most people are satisfied with this referral. But if there is another hospital close by that you and your parent like more, ask if the physician has privileges there as well. Many physicians have admitting privileges at more than one hospital.

When you have an option, you might want to do a little research on the hospital—especially if Mom or Dad has a condition that requires highly specialized care. Hospitals do go through an accreditation process supervised by the Joint Commission on Accreditation of Health Plans (JCAH), often referred to as the Joint Commission. Many states use the Joint Commission's review process instead of creating one on their own. The Joint Commission sends in a team of surveyors every three years to determine whether the hospital should be accredited. There are just over 5,100 hospitals in the United States. Here are the different "grades" they can get:

- **Accreditation with Commendation.** This is top-dog status. Only about 12 percent of hospitals have made this grade.

- **Accredited.** Approximately 4 percent of hospitals meet all the standards of care required to make this grade.

Senior Alert

Be aware that the Joint Commission is financially supported by the hospital industry. Critics feel that the accrediting system *by* hospitals *for* hospitals is a conflict of interest. Still, you should find out the hospital's status. You can also call your state Department of Health and ask for information on quality of care at hospitals.

- **Accredited with Recommendation for Improvement.** In this instance, hospitals have met most of the standards of care so they get accredited but there are a few things that they have to correct and are given a short period of time to turn them around. Most of the hospitals in this country—about 80 percent—fall into this category.

- **Provisional Accreditation, Conditional Accreditation, Preliminary Accreditation,** or **Non-accreditation.** If the hospital you are considering has any of these grades, then it's consumer beware. Find out why and start looking for other options. About 4 percent of hospitals have a negative accreditation status.

You can find out how well the hospital you're considering has performed on their latest Joint

Commission survey by calling 630-792-5800. They'll tell you the hospital's accreditation status and will send you a free copy of the report. You can also go to the Joint Commission's Web site at www.jcaho.org to receive the same information.

You and Mom might choose to travel to a specialized medical center, in which case her primary physician will need to make a referral to that institution. If Mom is in a Medicare HMO she *cannot* merrily go off and make this trip without prior approval by the HMO. If she does, it's at her expense! So make sure you know what hospitals and medical centers are covered by your parents' insurance before you entertain other options.

Arriving by Ambulance

You should become familiar with the terms of your parents' insurance policy on reimbursing for an ambulance trip in case of an emergency. Most Medi-gap policies and HMOs will also cover the rides *in an emergency.* The key here is what the insurance companies define as an emergency. Many states have laws that protect consumers if their insurance carriers refuse to reimburse the cost of the ambulance service or emergency room visit, if it turns out that Mom didn't have an emergency. For instance, say Mom's having chest pains and you think she's having a heart attack and call 911. After some pretty expensive tests, she's diagnosed with indigestion. That's the good news. The bad news? Because it wasn't a heart attack, and hence not an emergency, the insurance company doesn't pay. If this happens to your family, call your state Department of Health to find out what laws your state has passed that cover a layman's definition of emergency.

Sage Source

There are over 173 Veteran's Administration Hospitals throughout the country. If either of your parents qualifies, Mom or Dad may be eligible for care at one of these hospitals. You can find out what's available to your parents by calling 1-800-827-1000.

Consent at the Registration Desk

Several years ago, I needed neck surgery. My eyes couldn't get past "paralyzed from the neck down" as just *one* of the risks listed on the consent form. It is only right that hospitals lay out the cold, hard facts on the risks that any surgery or procedure presents. You and your parents need to weigh the benefits against the risks. No matter how minor the procedure, it isn't risk free!

Many people don't realize that they can make changes on the consent form. My surgery was performed at a very fine teaching hospital and I searched for the best neurosurgeon in my state. I wanted him to do the actual surgery and no one else.

I didn't mind other young doctors learning from him by being along side of him during the surgery. But that's where I wanted them to be: at his side. No scalpels in *their* hands. So on the section of the consent form where it said I gave permission for the surgery to the "surgeon or those under his supervision" I crossed out *or those under his supervision.* You can do the same.

If you have time to plan the hospital stay in advance, call the hospital and have them send you their blanket consent forms so that you can go over them.

If the hospital stay is unexpected, you could sign the form and simply write on the bottom, "I am signing this for admission purposes only." Once your parent has been admitted and you've had the time to look it over, then sign it.

Senior Alert

If your mom is having surgery, the other person critical to her care, other than her surgeon, is the anesthesiologist—the one who will put her to sleep and monitor her vital signs during surgery. Anesthesia is pretty tricky stuff, especially among the elderly. Ask about this person's credentials and arrange to be there during the face-to-face interview with your mom prior to surgery. You can also insist that the anesthesiologist not hand the job off to someone less qualified. There are also Nurse Anesthetists who are qualified to administer anesthesia. Make sure they are certified (CRNA). When your mom is "under," it's as close to death as she's ever going to be and still return—the anesthesiologist needs to know how close is close enough and how to bring her back!

Medical Errors in Hospitals

Here's a bulletin for you: Medical errors are one of the nation's leading causes of death and injury. The Institute of Medicine, a highly respected private, nonprofit group known for its health policy advice it gives Congress, recently reported that …

- Medical errors kill some 44,000 people in U.S. hospitals each year; however, another study said the number was closer to 98,000.
- More people die from medical mistakes each year than from highway accidents, breast cancer, or AIDS.
- Most of the medical errors are not the result of individual recklessness but from basic flaws in the way the health care system is organized. For example: illegible

handwriting of doctor's orders and stocking medicines at toxic, full-strength levels, which increases the risk for a hurried technician administering a toxic dose before remembering to dilute it.

- More than 7,000 people die each year both in and out of hospitals due to medication errors.

The Institute of Medicine's report has touched off quite a firestorm. The president of the United States and some members of congress claim that hospitals should be required to report all mistakes that cause serious injury and death. And hospitals should voluntarily report less serious errors including close calls. Right now, only about 18 states have laws demanding hospitals report medical errors, also known as adverse events.

So where does all this leave you and your parents? First you need to be an informed consumer and be as persistent as four-year-olds running around asking, "What's this?" and teenagers asking, "But, why?"

In the following sections I'll discuss the three most common areas of medical errors made in hospitals, along with steps you can take and questions you can ask so your parents don't become victims.

Infections

We all know that hospitals are places for very sick people, and very sick people have germs. Doctors, nurses, and technicians who care for these very sick people come in contact with them in the most intimate of ways: via blood, urine, and bodily contact. Germs happily jump on board any hospital staffer's hands and gain free access to every person with whom the staff person comes into contact—literally hundreds of people every day. Most of the patients have weakened immune systems, so they can't fight off all of the germs running rampant through the hospital. If they've had surgery, the site of the wound is a prime destination port for the germs. You don't need a Harvard medical degree to get the picture. The infections that people acquire in the hospital are known as *nosocomial infections.*

Geri-Fact

Nosocomial infections are hospital-acquired infections. They account for thousands of deaths and illnesses of people who have been hospitalized. Examples of these infections are pneumonia and bloodstream and urinary tract infections. The Centers for Disease Control report that nearly 88,000 deaths in 1995 were attributed to hospital-borne infections.

What can you and your parents do? Every hospital room has a bathroom with a sink and antibacterial soap. If you don't see the hospital employee or doctor go in and wash his or her hands, politely tell that person you'd feel much more comfortable if he or she would do so before touching your parent. If someone enters the room wearing gloves, ask that person to please put on a new pair. Make sure you, other family members, and friends wash their hands as soon as they've entered the room. And if anyone has a cold or flu—stay at home.

Senior Alert

If your parent comes down with an infection, ask the doctor for the exact name and spelling of the infection. Also ask to see someone from the Infection Control Unit (every hospital must have one). Ask for an explanation of the nature of the infection, and what the best practices are to treat it. You should also ask for the hospital's infection rate. If this infection has caused a real hardship for your parent, report the incident to your local health department. You may prevent somebody else's Mom or Dad from going through the same thing.

Physician Error

Whenever I was furious with my little brother who had just toppled over my Lincoln Log house (okay, so I predate Legos), my grandmother would intervene and say, "To err is human but to forgive is divine." Well, I wasn't feeling too divine at eight years old but the point sank in as the years rolled on. Doctors have been given pretty divine status in this culture, so it comes as quite a surprise and disappointment when they make a mistake. And doctors *do* make mistakes.

Here are a few things you can do to safeguard your parent from physician error:

- When it comes to surgery, always ask for a second opinion. This is something that you'll probably have to push for because many of our parents' generation think second opinions are an insult to their doctors, but many physicians welcome another doc's opinion. If there is another, safer way to treat Mom or Dad's condition without surgery, it's definitely worth researching.

- Make your own allergies alert notice by writing down the drugs your parent is allergic to and taping it on the head of Mom or Dad's bed. Also write down any medical conditions your parent has (diabetes, for example).

- Immediately report to the doctor and nurse any side effects your parent experiences with the drugs he or she is taking.

- Over-the-counter drugs still count as drugs. Don't give your parent his or her usual dose of aspirin or even vitamins without checking with the doctor.

- Bring to the hospital the list of drugs your mom or dad is taking. Review these with the doctor to determine what your parent should continue taking during the hospital stay. Be sure to ask the doctor about any complications that can arise if new drugs are added to the regimen. The more drugs you parent is taking, the more likely he or she is going to run into complications from adverse drug interactions.

Geri-Fact

Many errors in hospitals involve giving the wrong medication, the wrong dosage, or medication that the patient is allergic to—even though the correct information is stated on patients' charts. Get Mom or Dad to always ask the name of the drugs when a nurse hands your parent pills to take. Your parents should know both the brand and generic name of the drugs they're allergic to so they'll recognize either name. Mom or Dad should always ask what medication is being pumped through an intravenous line and what it's supposed to do. If your parent isn't able to ask these questions, *you* ask. Always!

Bed Sores

Your parents' skin becomes more fragile with age. Laying in one position for long periods of time can irritate their sensitive skin, especially in bony areas such as the heels, elbows, and tail bone where pressure decreases the blood flow. Sometimes you'll hear the term "pressure sores" rather than bed sores for this reason. If Mom isn't being routinely repositioned or "turned" as it is commonly referred to, her skin begins to get red and tender. If not treated immediately, an open wound will develop which becomes a prime source for infections. These are especially feared in nursing homes, but I have seen patients with very good skin condition come back to the nursing home from a hospital stay with several pressure sores because no one took the time to routinely turn them. So be sure to check over Mom's sensitive spots and make sure she's being repositioned. Ask the staff to provide an egg-crate foam mattress, which are used to prevent pressure sores, to put on top of the hospital bed mattress. Be sure to take it home with you.

Becoming a Patient Advocate

There are people at the hospital with this title. If you have a problem or a conflict with anyone or any policy of the hospital system, ask to see the patient advocate because he or she can be very helpful in assisting you in reaching a solution. But the best advocacy for your parents comes from you. Here's how to become their *personal* patient advocate:

1. Get to know the nurses at the nurse's station. Introduce yourself and choose one or two family members who will be the liaison with other family members to give updates on Mom or Dad's condition. Don't bombard the nurses or make a nuisance of yourself.

2. Ask the nurses how you can help out (for example, getting fluids for Mom, helping her get in and out of bed, taking Dad for his daily exercise down the hall either by wheelchair or walking, taking Mom to and from the bathroom or helping Dad use the urinal. Of course, you can do these things only if you are able and it's safe for you to do so. But offering this kind of help is greatly appreciated by the staff.

3. Educate yourself on your mom or dad's condition so that you can have an informed discussion with the physician when you need to discuss treatment options.

4. Don't be afraid to insist on seeing the doctor or at the very least, to get him or her on the phone. Many doctors make their rounds very early in the morning, so ask the nurses when the doc is due in and make it a point to be there. If you can't because of work, tell them you want an appointment.

5. If you disagree with the doctor or the insurance plan's decision to withhold treatment (such as not giving your parent physical therapy), ask to speak to a representative of the hospital's medical or ethics committee. Tell the representative you want to know how to appeal the decision.

6. If the Medicare HMO refuses a procedure or admission, or you think Dad is being discharged too soon, get to the patient advocate

Sage Source

If your parent is on Medicare, you have another resource: In every state there is a peer review organization (PRO). The PRO consists of a group of physicians working for the federal government who go over complaints and decide whether the action cited in the complaint was in the patient's best interest. Hospitals must give you information on how to contact your PRO. To reach the PRO, call the Office of Medical Review at 410-966-6851 or your area agency on aging.

at the hospital and find out the steps you need to take to reverse the decision. Every HMO must provide you a number to call to appeal a decision, so get that number. Sometimes, just making an inquiry can get Mom that extra day she might need.

7. There is a major nursing shortage in this country, and hospitals have been forced to use temporary agencies that send in registered nurses who might not be familiar with the hospital's routine and procedures. Hospitals might also use nursing assistants who are not as well trained as registered nurses to identify troubling symptoms following surgery. Don't assume that someone wearing white is a full-fledged nurse or doctor. Ask for the name of the registered nurse (RN) assigned to monitor your parent during each shift. Make sure each one is personally checking over your parent's care.

Trust Your Instincts

I remember when my Dad had surgery, an aide took him down the hall for his first walk. He looked pale to me. She asked him if everything was okay. I knew he wouldn't complain, so she kept encouraging him to walk. But I intervened and said I thought he should go back to bed. Once he was back in bed, I noticed his breathing seemed shallow and his color hadn't returned. I called in the nurse and told her something was wrong, although I could tell she clearly thought I was over reacting. I finally insisted that the doctor see him. Turns out he was rushed to intensive care because the doctor discovered an air bubble (emboli) in his lung. Had he continued walking, it could have burst and he would have died. Remember, I'm not a physician or nurse—I just knew my Dad. So, don't be afraid to express your concerns and quickly go up the ladder to make them known. Trust your instincts!

If You Can't Be There

If you or your siblings absolutely can't be there during your parent's hospital stay, make sure you talk once a day with the nurse and doctor in charge of your parent's care. If you can afford it, hire a private duty nurse or nurse's aide to take your place. If you have siblings, decide among you who is the "point guard" with the doctors and nurses. All of you shouldn't be calling. If necessary, organize a conference call with the doctor and your siblings if very critical decisions have to be made. Make sure arrangements are made to provide your parent with care when he or she gets home. Home health care agencies are very good at letting you know how things are going with your parent every time they look in on them. See the next chapter for details on home health care.

Home Sweet Home

You're probably thinking, "Hey, my dad just got here and you want to discharge him already?" Every hospital has a department dedicated to discharge planning. This is usually a group of social workers who can assist you and your parents in making plans to go home. The deal here, however, is for you to make sure that it's prudent for your parent to go home, especially if Mom or Dad lives alone or will go home to an ailing spouse. If you need to bring in help, review the personal care aide section in Chapter 10, "Home Health Care."

Geri-Fact

Medicare pays about 40 percent of all the hospital bills in this country so they're rightly concerned about the high cost of medical care. To keep costs under control, Medicare figured out the average cost of hundreds of procedures and categorized these into diagnostic related groups (DRGs). The hospital's financial interest is to get your parents in and out of the hospital without going over the amount it's going to get under the DRG. In fact, if the hospital discharges patients sooner, the hospital pockets the money. So don't let the hospital shorten the stay when your parent isn't able to go home. (See "Becoming a Patient Advocate" earlier in this chapter.)

There's nothing your parents will like more than crawling under the covers of their very own bed, but sooner or later they'll have to poke their heads out and face the inevitable hospital bills.

Medicare statements start rolling in and they usually begin with *This Is Not a Bill*. My take on this is that they're just trying to prevent heart attacks. At some point, they start becoming bills and you get them from the hospital's laboratory, the surgeons, the anesthesiologists, and all kinds of therapists. The hospital bill will probably list a zillion codes and the costs will seem out of sight. Since Medicare will cover 80 percent of the bill, most hospitals mark up the price so that the 80 percent really covers what they consider is 100 percent of their costs. Under Medicare Part A your parents pay a one-time deductible and the other 20 percent if they don't have a Medi-gap policy. Bottom line? Make sure they have one!

And here's something else to keep in mind: According to the U.S. General Accounting Office, almost all hospital bills contain mistakes! Before you pay any out-of-pocket expenses (besides the mandatory Medicare deductible), ask for an itemized bill from the hospital's billing department. This is the only way you can determine if your parents were billed for the same procedure twice, if they were billed for a procedure they didn't get, or catch something that just looks wrong. Besides getting the hospital's mail, Mom and Dad will be hearing from their Medi-gap policy buddies who are picking up the tab for the 20 percent Medicare didn't pay. They might get separate bills from the doctor's office who treated them. Some states have passed legislation that doesn't allow doctors to charge more than what Medicare covers. You'll need to find out if your state has passed this legislation. Your local area agency on aging (see Appendix B, "National List of State Units on Aging.") can tell you.

Sage Source

Representatives of the Seniors Health Insurance Program (SHIP) can help you sort through your Medicare bills and tell you who covers what. They can also show you how to appeal denials. Call you local area agency on aging or senior center to find out how to contact a SHIP representative. You can also call the National Insurance Consumer Helpline at 1-800-942-4242.

The Least You Need to Know

- Chances are your parent will need a hospital stay in the near future. If you have the option, do some research on the hospital before your parent needs to be admitted.

- You can alter consent forms for surgery and hospital stays to give your parents added protection. Take the time to read them carefully.

- With over 44,000 people dying of medical errors in hospitals each year, you need to protect your parent from becoming a casualty.

- Become your mom or dad's personal patient advocate by taking steps such as educating yourself on your parent's condition so you can discuss treatment options with the doctor.

- If you can't be with your mom or dad during his or her hospital stay, there are still things you and your siblings can do to keep in touch with the situation.

- According to the U.S. Government Accounting Office, most hospitals bills contain errors. Ask for an itemized bill from the hospital and look it over carefully.

Home Health Care

When Grandma, at age 95, came to live with us she was suffering from dementia resulting from malnutrition. She had wanted to live alone but stopped eating because she thought her food was poisoned. Following her cataract surgery, good nutrition, and lots of love, she made a terrific recovery. She enjoyed getting out and going to adult day care. (She had a crush on her exercise teacher.) Whenever anyone wanted to do anything with her, she would tell them they would have to check with her "manager"—me. We had quite a year together. My most treasured moment was when she greeted me at the door when I brought our infant son home. His room was next to his great grandma's.

Then Grandma started having strokes. Each one took their toll. And each one took me through the same maze of health care that I'll share with you in this chapter.

What Does Your Parent Need?

There are basically three different levels of care that come under the heading of home health care: homemaker services, home health care, and skilled care. The first thing you'll need to do is determine what your parent needs, and then search for the level of care that fits Mom or Dad's needs.

Homemaker Care

Perhaps Dad needs help with what geriatricians call the *instrumental* activities of daily living, such as …

- Meal preparation
- Heavy housework
- Doing the laundry
- Grocery shopping
- Managing money
- Keeping track of medications
- Getting around in the community via personal or public transportation

Senior Alert

When it comes to managing money, keep as much of this responsibility in your hands as possible. Even if you have to do this from a distance, have Dad's Social Security and pension checks electronically deposited into his bank account. Use a bill payer service with a bank to have all of his routine bills paid electronically. If you live far away, have the home care aide mail you any nonroutine bills so that you can pay them. Be extremely careful handing off money matters to strangers or friends.

If Dad needs this kind of help, it might make sense to hire a homemaker or chore worker to prepare meals, remind Dad to take his medicines properly (the worker is not permitted to administer medications, however), handle the grocery shopping, keep up with the laundry, and perhaps take him to doctor appointments or to social events. For these kinds of things, Dad doesn't need anyone with a nursing background to care for him. The focus here is on providing care for your dad to live at home; in other words, *home care.*

This level of care can prevent your dad from needing more extensive care down the line. Getting someone in, even two days a week, can prevent Dad from eating poorly, forgetting to take his medicine, and not attending to his physical hygiene. It doesn't always take a catastrophic event to send Dad down a fast descent. Malnutrition can lead to dementia, mixing up medicines can easily land him in the hospital, and poor hygiene can lead to infections.

Home Health Care Aide

If your mom needs help with activities of daily living that are more physical in nature, then you need to move up a level on the home health care ladder. Perhaps your mom needs help with the following:

- Eating
- Dressing
- Bathing
- Using the toilet
- Getting in and out of bed
- Taking medications
- Getting around inside of the home

If Mom needs help doing these things, a home health care aide who has some training in health care (such as a certified nurse's aide) would be the best bet. You might hear the term *custodial* care or *personal* care being used to describe the kind of services your mom needs.

Senior Alert

Giving a bath to an older person is no easy matter. Knowing how to move someone without you or the other person falling is a trained skill. If you hire someone to give Mom or Dad a bath, ask that person about his or her training, particularly how he or she avoids falls in the bathroom.

The certified nurse's aide would do well to be supervised by a nurse on a periodic basis. The nurse's role would be to set up a care plan, monitor the plan and Mom's condition, and identify any other potential problems that may arise. A nurse is best prepared to pick up symptoms that warrant further examination by a physician. If you're working with an agency, most will have a nurse oversee the care provided by a nurse's aide.

Skilled Care

The level of home care requires skilled nursing care. In this instance, registered nurses (RNs) or licensed practical nurses (LPNs) provide direct, hands-on nursing care to your mom or dad. This is usually needed following surgery or recuperation from a stroke. Besides needing most of the custodial care just discussed, Mom or Dad may need dressings changed, medications administered, and various therapies provided.

At this level, a doctor prescribes the kind of care that your parent should receive. The doctor might also order physical therapy, occupational therapy, speech therapy, or respiratory therapy. A nurse will oversee the care being provided by all of these therapists and nurse's aides.

Searching for Providers

You can go down two different paths in your search for home health care: hire someone on your own or go through an agency. If you hire someone on your own, then take the time to research that person's background to protect your parent. There are plenty of horror stories about how older people have had their life savings stolen or the care was so poor that they ended up in a life-threatening situation.

Finding Your Own Health Care Worker: Hiring Tips

- Describe your mom or dad's condition(s) and ask the worker to describe what he or she would do for your parent.
- Ask the worker to tell you what training he or she has had for each task described.
- Ask the worker to show you any certificates or educational degrees he or she has received.
- Ask for a resume that identifies the school the worker attended, previous jobs, and names of employers.
- If your parent suffers from dementia, find out what specialized training the worker has received to meet Mom or Dad's needs?
- What training has the worker had in lifting people? Is this person able to meet the physical demands of your parent?
- Ask the worker to provide you with a copy of the results of a police background check.
- Ask for a list of references—and then call them! Make sure that at least two references are from families who have used the worker's services.

The first step is to find a referral source you can trust. You can call a local senior center, a faith-based organization, the area agency on aging, social workers at any local hospital, or your doctor's office. These sources might know of someone who is very reputable. Consider the following tips in your employment venture.

It's a good idea to interview prospective employees at a neutral place, like a local coffee shop. This way you are not exposing your parent's vulnerability or home to perfect strangers. Once you have narrowed down your search, invite your top two picks (after you've called references) to the home and see how they interact with your parent.

If you are hiring a certified nurse's aide, you can also check with your State Department of Health and ask if they maintain the nurse's aide registry required by federal law. Ask how you can check to see if the nurse's aide you are about to employ has been reported for any wrongdoing.

Hiring Through a Home Health Care Agency

If you decide to hire someone through an agency, you do gain some added protections that you don't when you go it alone. The first thing you want to find out is if the agency is certified by a state or federal agency. If the agency receives reimbursements from Medicaid (state) or Medicare (federal) then it has to meet legislated standards of care and safety regulations. People who are employed by the agency meet certain training criteria. The agency should also be paying for workers' compensation in the event a worker becomes injured on the job. This reduces your liability. Chances are the agency is bonded so that any damage caused by an employee will be covered by the agency. You also have a greater opportunity to track the performance record of the agency than you do a private citizen's. Here's a list of questions you should ask when approaching an agency:

Geri-Fact

If you hire someone on your own, you will probably save money. However, you are responsible for paying for the employee's Social Security and Medicare taxes if you pay the worker $1,200 or more in cash during the year. To know the full details on how to pay and report wages, check out Social Security's Web site at www.ssa.gov and enter the keywords Household Workers on the search bar.

> ## Going Through a Home Health Care Agency: What to Ask
>
> - Does Medicaid or Medicare certify the agency?
> - Is the agency accredited by any professional organization?
> - What state licenses does the agency have? What has been its compliance record over the last two years?
> - Is the agency bonded? Are all employees covered?
> - What kind of background check does the agency conduct on all of its employees?
> - What services does the agency provide? What are the costs?
> - Does the agency conduct an assessment to determine my parent's needs? Who conducts the assessment? (Make sure it's at least a registered nurse.)
> - How does the agency work with my parent's primary doctor?
> - Who coordinates my parent's care? What level of training does that person have?
> - How much of the paperwork does the agency handle for third-party payments (insurance, Medicare, Medicaid)?
> - Does the agency offer 24-hour availability in case of any emergency?
> - Does the agency provide immediate backup should one of its workers not show up?
> - Can we get a replacement if the worker does not do well with my parent?
> - Are there certain things your workers are *not* allowed to do?
> - Is there a minimum number of hours we have to contract with you to receive the service?

Who's Who in the Home Health Care Biz

As with so much these days, nothing's simple. With so many people being able to be cared for at home with the rise of durable medical equipment and *infusion therapy*, you'll run into a number of different professions and companies. Here are the basics.

Senior Alert

You may hear the term *registry* when you look for home health care. Registries are employment agencies for home care nurses and aides. They match up the workers with families requesting the service and collect finder's fees from the workers. These agencies are not licensed or regulated, nor are they required to conduct background checks of the people they refer to you. If you employ someone from a registry, you are responsible for paying all taxes and following all labor, health, and safety laws and regulations. Don't assume that someone referred to you by a registry has met any licensing or training requirements. These are *not* certified home health care agencies.

Durable Medical Equipment (DME) and Supply Companies

These companies provide home care patients products and supplies ranging from respirators, wheelchairs, walkers, and hospital beds to catheters and wound care supplies. Many of these companies will deliver the equipment to your home and many handle the paperwork with Medicare. Dealers who bill Medicare must meet minimum federal standards, and some states require these companies to be licensed. They are listed in the Yellow Pages.

Pharmaceutical and Infusion Therapy Companies

These companies deliver medications, equipment, and professional services to people who are receiving intravenous (IV) or nutritional therapies through specially placed tubes. Nutrition infusion therapy helps individuals who cannot be sustained through normal feeding because of a permanent malfunction of their digestive system. Other forms of infusion therapy provide chemotherapy, administration of morphine for cancer patients, and infusion pumps to treat other conditions. Medicare covers infusion therapy only if a physician has submitted a signed Certification of Medical Necessity. Home infusion therapy providers

Geri-Fact

Infusion therapy is what most of us think of when we're hooked up to an IV (intravenous) line in the hospital. The IV is one type of infusion therapy. Medications are being infused into your body. There is a wide variety of infusion pumps, supplies, and equipment (besides an IV) that infuse nutrition, medications, and chemotherapy into patients. All of these fall under the term infusion therapy.

Sage Source

For more information about home health care, contact the National Association for Home Care, 228 Seventh Street S.E., Washington, DC 20003; 202-547-7424. Their Web site (www.nahc.org) offers a Home Care and Hospice Locator and an online guide on how to choose a home care provider. Or contact the Visiting Nurse Association of America, 3801 East Florida Avenue, Suite 900, Denver, CO 80210; 1-800-426-2547 or www.vnaa.org.

must meet certain standards to receive a Medicare supplier number. Make sure that you deal only with an agency certified by Medicare. The companies employ pharmacists who prepare solutions and nurses who show patients how to take the medications and nutritional therapies. Some states require these agencies to be licensed.

The Cast of Therapists

Your parent might be prescribed a number of different therapists by his or her physician:

- **Physical therapists** (**PTs**) restore the mobility and strength of patients who are limited or disabled, oftentimes as a result of strokes. Through exercise, massage, and equipment PTs alleviate pain and restore functioning. They also teach families and patients how to transfer from chairs, beds, and toilets. These therapists are licensed and have post-graduate education and training.

- **Occupational therapists** (**OTs**) help your parent perform the activities of daily living (eating, bathing, using the toilet, cooking, dressing, and doing basic household chores). They can assess the home and identify ways to make living at home easier and safer. OTs can show your parent how to use adaptive equipment and devices to make everyday life easier. OTs have received special training and are also licensed.

- **Speech language pathologists** help your parent restore his or her speech if it's lost or if Dad or Mom become disabled in his or her ability to communicate due to strokes, surgery, or injury.

  These therapists can also help them with breathing, swallowing, and muscle control. These individuals are licensed and have post-graduate training beyond college.

- **Registered dieticians** (**RDs**) assist your parent and professional staff in developing a nutritional plan for your parent given certain medical conditions. They are licensed following post-graduate training.

- **Respiratory therapists** (**RTs**) evaluate, treat, and care for patients with breathing disorders. They operate sophisticated equipment to administer oxygen, manage mechanical ventilation for people who can't breathe on their own, administer medications in aerosol form, and manage overall therapy to help patients breathe better. There are two levels of respiratory therapists: the certified therapist and registered therapist. RTs are required to have either an associate's degree (two years of college) or a four-year college degree in the sciences. They may take a national voluntary exam to become a Certified Respiratory Therapist (CRT). They can also take two more exams to become a Registered Respiratory Therapist (RRT).

Who Pays for What?

There are five major sources of payment for home health care: self-pay, Medicare, Medicaid, insurance, and community service programs.

1. Medicare usually covers your mom or dad's home health care if your parent is homebound, under a physician's care, and requires medically necessary skilled nursing or therapy services. A physician must order these services for Mom or Dad. Medical equipment and supplies along with different therapies are also covered under the Medicare home health benefit. The services must be intermittent, meaning part-time. The rules governing home health care benefits change frequently, so check in often with the Web site at www.medicare.gov. You can track down the home health care intermediary's phone number for your region at the site.

2. Medicaid is a joint state-federal medical assistance program for people with low incomes. Because Medicaid is state administered, each state has its own rules and benefits governing home health care benefits. The best way to determine if your parent qualifies for programs in your state is to contact the local area agency on aging (see Appendix B, "National List of State Units on Aging") or your local welfare office.

3. Various insurance programs will cover home health care but you really have to read your policies well. Some Medi-gap policies offer at-home recovery services when the policyholder is receiving Medicare-covered skilled home health services, but it must be ordered by your mom or dad's physician. This type of coverage is often used to help your parent recover from surgery or an acute illness.

Senior Alert

Home health agencies must give you a notice that explains why and when they estimate Medicare will stop paying for your mom or dad's home health care. If you believe your parent needs continued home health care, you can appeal the decision. Ask the home health care agency for the 800 number of the regional home health intermediary. If you want to take the risk, you can still receive home care services and pay the agency directly. If you win the appeal, Medicare will reimburse you.

Long-term care insurance policies also offer home health care services but plans vary widely with different sets of requirements. If your mom or dad has such a plan, read it carefully *before* bringing in home health care services.

4. Medicare managed care plans must offer the same exact benefit that original Medicare provides. Some plans offer more than Medicare; again, read the policies carefully.

5. The Veterans Administration will provide home health care services to veterans who are at least 50 percent disabled due to a service-related condition. A physician must authorize the service, and the care is delivered through the VA's hospital-based home care units. Homemaker services are not covered.

Community organizations do offer a number of home health care services to assist families' care for a loved one at home. Some states offer family caregiver support programs through their area agency on aging. Faith-based groups offer companion services and homemaker services, and some home health care agencies offer care at reduced rates for low-income persons. Check with the area agency on aging to find out what's available in your community and state.

Setting Up Ground Rules

If you hire through an agency, the agency usually provides the staff with a set of ground rules that they are to follow. Ask to see those rules so that you'll understand what is expected of them. By working with a home health care agency, you also have the advantage of having a supervisor whom you can turn to if problems arise. However, do try to work out differences *before* you go to a worker's supervisor.

Make a list of Mom's routines and special preferences that you want considered as part of her care plan. Perhaps she has a certain breakfast at a certain time every morning (Grandma and I had tea and toast every morning at 9:00 A.M.) or wears a particular robe when she's about to take a bath and turns on the space heater 15 minutes before bath time. She might be on a diabetic diet or be on a set schedule for using the toilet. Put all of this in writing, so that every worker will be following the same guidelines. Having a set routine is comforting to most older people. Don't brush it aside.

Besides your parent's care routine, you'll need to let the worker know how much of the house they

Silver Lining

Working with frail, elderly people, especially those with dementia, can be very trying. Say thank you to those providing care to your parent. Show them through little extras—small gifts, their favorite food, and some private space—how much you appreciate what they are doing. Make them feel part of a very special circle of family and friends.

will have access to. There may be certain rooms that are considered off limits, such as other bedrooms. Usually the kitchen becomes a communal space where you can offer the worker space in the refrigerator for lunch or dinner and access to the microwave. It's also wise to inform the worker that friends and family members are not permitted to visit while he or she is on the job.

The more you clarify expectations from the start, the more likely you and your parent will develop a positive and nurturing relationship with your home health care worker. On the other hand, don't go overboard with the list so that the worker feels overwhelmed and not very welcomed. You are hiring a health care worker for his or her professional services and caring attitude. This person, too, needs to feel at home with your family.

Nurturing a Relationship

Your parents need to feel respected and valued by those caring for them. Mom may feel resentful that she's losing her independence and that she has to rely on strangers for such private things as bathing and using the toilet, so she may act out her frustration on others. Those who care for her will need to be patient and sensitive. It will be easier for them to be patient if they get to know your mom as a person. So take out the family photo album, and show them pictures of Mom in her younger days: what kind of work she did, her volunteer projects, the kids she's raised, the man she married, her hobbies and interests. Also let them know what kind of things "gets her goat" or any hot buttons that could get them on the wrong foot with your mom. And I'm sure there are some things that could win favor with Mom pretty quickly, too. Don't keep them a secret.

Take the time to get to know new members of your team that cares for your parent. Learn about *their* interests and hobbies so that you can share those with your mom while introductions are underway. Hopefully, they'll find something in common to begin this new relationship. If you live far away, encourage the home health care aide or nurse to call you frequently to update you on Mom's care. You may also need to be involved to help smooth things over and keep the communication channels open.

Sage Source

If you suspect elder abuse, neglect, or financial exploitation, call the elder abuse hotline of your area agency on aging found in the Yellow Pages. You can call the Eldercare Locator at 1-800-677-1116 to find the area agency on aging closest to you. All calls are kept in strictest confidence. The area agency on aging has the professional training to detect and determine what's really going on. By law they must respond to your complaint quickly.

Be Careful

As with every profession, there are always some bad apples. Protect yourself by keeping jewelry and money out of sight from employees. Your parent shouldn't have large sums of cash stowed away somewhere in the house. If your parent has a liquor cabinet, keep it locked or get rid of it if it's no longer being used. Never hand over bank accounts or ATM cards to workers. If you live in the area, drop in once in awhile unannounced. If you live far away, ask a trusted neighbor to be your eyes and ears.

Always watch for unexplained bruises or reports that your parent keeps falling because these could be signs of abuse. Watch how medications are being used, too. If your parent is prescribed pain pills, be alert to frequent refills being ordered; this could point to drug abuse by the worker (or even by Dad). If Dad becomes extremely withdrawn around the worker, or shows other behavior that is out of character for him, talk with him. Perhaps something is going on and he's afraid to bring it up. If he complains—more than usual—talk with the worker or the worker's supervisor. Don't jump to conclusions, because there are stages of Alzheimer's where people can become very paranoid. However, you should talk with your dad's physician to determine how much of Dad's fears are real. Even if his fears are not substantiated, you might consider finding a replacement, because your dad's emotional comfort is vital to his well-being.

The Least You Need to Know

- There are three levels of home care: homemaker services, home health care, and skilled care.

- You have more protection and assurances of quality care if you work with a Medicare-certified home health care agency. Be careful of hiring people from registries; these are *not* certified home health care agencies.

- If you decide to hire someone on your own, check out references, verify training certificates, and ask for a copy of a police background check.

- Medicare will cover home health care services only if your parent is homebound and a physician says it's absolutely necessary.

- Routine is comforting to most older people. Be sure to write out the routine of care that your parent needs and expects and share it with the health care worker.

- If you suspect your parent is being abused or neglected by a home health care worker, contact your local area on agency (1-800-677-1116) or call their Elder Abuse Hotline listed in the blue pages of your phone book.

Part 3

Understanding You and Your Parents' Options

Far too many older people think that there are only two choices in their retirement years: live at home or take up residence in a nursing home. But "home sweet home" can take many forms as your parents age. If they do want to stay at home, there are all kinds of ways to make independent living safe, affordable, and senior-friendly. In this part you'll be given the keys to unlock services like home-delivered meals, insurance, health screenings, and transportation. We'll also help you assess whether or not it's time for your parent to turn in those car keys.

Besides all of the independent ways of living, your parents might do better in a continuing care retirement community or at an assisted living facility. You'll learn about the differences, and how to assess the best place for your parents. And if your mom or dad needs a nursing home, we'll show you how to find a quality home and, once your parents are living there, how to make your visits count.

Remaining at Home: Making It Work

As members of the GI generation of WWII, your mom and dad experienced the American dream of homeownership more than any other generation before or after them. Owning a home represented the good life and they fully expected to raise their families and visit with their grandchildren in the same home. To further add to their rooted lifestyle, many men enjoyed jobs with the same employer for their entire work life.

So, it should be no surprise to you that your parents want to stay at home for as long as they can. But as your parents age and become more frail, the quest for independence may tip the scales against safety. It's one of the hardest issues you, as their child, are going to face. How much do you honor your parents' need for independence without compromising their safety?

Home *Safe* Home

There are a number of things you can do to tip the scales in your parents' favor for safely living at home. The ideas and strategies I'm going to share with you will work for both parents, Dad or Mom. But because I've received so many calls over the years from friends trying to struggle with their mother's decision to live alone, this chapter will focus on Mom. But of course, the strategies apply to either parent.

The operative word here is *decision*. Don't think you're doing Mom a favor by picking out new digs for her to live. She also might not be hot on the idea of living with you—even if you have the room and all the resources in the world to accommodate her. To give up her space represents much more than bricks and mortar. It means acknowledging that she's not the independent go-getter she used to be and that she's vulnerable—to falling and no one being there to help, or falling prey to people who'll take advantage of her. None of this is too easy to accept. So don't go rushing in to fix things and take control. It's control your mom is worried about losing. So let's find ways to reinforce her sense of control and make her safe.

Outside Safety

The first thing you want to do is make sure Mom's surroundings are safe, so that she doesn't start confining herself to the house because she's afraid to go outside or come home in the dark. Make it a point to come home with her in the early evening to better identify her safety concerns and needs. Think of the things that would make you feel safer. Here are a few ideas:

- **Motion-sensitive lighting.** Perhaps it's time to install new lights that automatically turn on when there's any movement near them. For any would-be intruders, an automatic light outside the entryway tells them someone is at home and is aware that they are in the driveway. The other advantage is that, even if Mom forgets to turn on the lights before she left during the day, the light will be on for her when she comes home.

- **Lights on timers.** Mom should also have timers for outside lights and a light in the bathroom to turn them on and keep them on throughout the night so that anyone casing the house will think someone is up. Timers are an inexpensive way to burglar-proof the house. They are installed by simply plugging them into an electrical outlet.

- **Keys and the neighbors.** If your mom lives in the old neighborhood where you grew up you may still know the neighbors. If not, when you visit her get to know a couple of her neighbors. If she's living in a high-rise, get to know the security people (if there aren't any security guards, meet the neighbors across the hall). The purpose of getting to know the neighbors is to identify someone that you *and* your mom trust to have an extra set of keys to her house. Share phone numbers so that if either of you becomes concerned about Mom—she hasn't answered the phone or the mail is piling up—you can call each other and the neighbor can look in on her.

- **Getting into the house.** If your mom drives and has a garage but no automatic garage-door opener, now would be a good time to get one. If you have siblings to help with the cost, the opener can become very affordable if all of you pitch in. There are also systems available that turn on a radio a few minutes before Mom enters the house so that the noise can alert a burglar to run rather than be surprised and possibly hurt Mom as he attempts to escape. Wherever she parks the car should be well lit, which can also be controlled by remote control as she enters the driveway. Make sure the pathway to and from the house is clear of any obstacles so that Mom won't trip over them. If bushes create a good hiding place for an attacker, trim them or relocate them to another part of the yard. Mom should always ask taxi drivers and her friends to please wait until they see her enter the house.

Senior Alert

Never hide a house key outside the house, even in one of those cute turtle statues or fake rocks, and certainly not under the mat or flowerpot. Burglars are far too aware of where we "clever" homeowners hide our keys. Consider installing a keyless lock (available at any hardware store). Of course, the neighbors will need to know the code and your mom must be able to remember it.

- **Friendly local police.** Most communities throughout the country have local police who will drive by Mom's neighborhood as a security measure, if you ask. You should also find out from the local police if there is a neighborhood watch group in her neighborhood and let the group know she lives alone, and that you'd appreciate it if they kept an eye out for her.

- **Friendly postal carriers and utility meter readers.** Most mail carriers work the same route every day and get to know a neighborhood quite well. The U.S. Postal Service has a program to alert the area agency on aging if the carrier believes there is a problem. Utility companies do the same. Call thelocal area agency on aging to find out if this program exists in your community (1-800-677-1116) .

- **Security systems.** If you can afford it, investing in a security system not only protects your mom but also provides her with peace of mind. You'll need to make sure, however, that she can easily operate the system so that she's not constantly triggering the alarms. Be sure to be part of this decision so that she isn't sold something more complicated or extensive than what she needs. And don't forget the simple things, like installing a peephole in the front and side doors, a deadbolt, and an intercom so she won't have to open the door to a stranger.

Inside Safety

"I've fallen and I can't get up." What most people fear when living alone is that something will happen to them—a fall, a stroke, a heart attack—and they won't be able to get to a phone to call for help. If this is of great concern to your mom or she has a condition that raises the likelihood that such a situation could occur, look into getting a personal medical alert system. These systems offer your parent a choice of wearing a necklace with a pendant on it or a bracelet like a watchband. If there's an emergency, all they need to do is push a button and it will alert an emergency responder who will send in an emergency crew. Some systems are able to activate an intercom on Mom's phone to ask her what is wrong and then call a responder.

There are several different systems out there, so do your research. Some charge for the devices separately while others include it in their monthly service fee (similar to cell phone contracts that include the phone). The most important thing you need to know is the capability of the answering service. Be sure to ask …

Geri-Fact

Personal medical alert systems can be found in the Yellow Pages under Medical Alarms. You can also ask your family doctor, local hospital, or medical supply store for a referral. Some companies will sell you a system where you buy the equipment. This can become pretty expensive, costing upward of $2,000. Most people pay a monthly fee of around $50 month.

- What kind of training has the staff who receive the calls had?
- What formal relationships does the service have with the local emergency response services in the community?
- If English is a second language for your mom, does the service have an interpreter?
- What is the company's average response time?
- Is there a trial period for the service?

Be sure to test the system once Mom brings it home to determine its range throughout the house and how far she can use it outdoors such as to the mailbox.

Creating a Senior-Friendly Home

When I was caring for my son while his great grandmother lived with us, I led a rather schizophrenic life. At one end of the house I was creating obstacles to keep him *out* of trouble and at the other end of the house I was taking away obstacles to keep Grandma from getting *into* trouble.

Today, there are many things you can do to make your mom's home a safer, more user-friendly place to make the quality of her life better and easier. Here are some of my top picks.

Dining in: The Kitchen

Believe it or not, one in four people over 65 years of age is malnourished. Cooking for one seems to discourage older people from making a healthy meal. They also find opening jars, fidgeting with the stove, and reaching for pots and pans a hassle. Here are some ways to make life in the kitchen easier and safer:

- Encourage Mom to use a microwave oven to prevent accidents on gas or electric ranges.

- Replace standard dials on the stove with easy-to-read, large dials. Make sure the off button is very visible (consider marking it red).

- Take a look at Mom's small appliances. Do they need to be updated? Make sure she has an easy, automatic can opener, a jar opener, a small microwave that can be easily programmed for her favorite meals, and a toaster oven to heat meals.

- Hang potholders near the stove for easy access so Mom won't have a need to grab a towel or use an apron. Advise her not to wear housecoats or other apparel with large open sleeves that can get caught on the stove or pot handle.

- Make use of lazy Susans so that dishes, pots, pans, and cooking materials Mom uses most frequently are in easy reach so she isn't reaching too high or too low which can throw her off balance.

- Invest in a set of clear-plastic microwavable containers for heating and storing small portions of food.

Sage Source

There are all kinds of gadgets to make cooking easier that are available through catalogs, on-line, and at specialty stores at the mall. The National Rehab Information Center (1-800-346-2742) offers information on products for easy living for people with disabilities. Or contact the Access Foundation at 516-568-2715.

Danger Zone: The Bathroom

Here's a room where you really need to invest some energy and make some changes. More accidents occur in this room than in any other space in the house. Here's what you can do:

- Place rubber, nonskid strips on the bathroom floor and nonskid bathmats in the tub and/or shower.

- If Mom uses a shower, make sure the shower curtain is not held up by a tension rod—if she grabs it for support, she'll fall with it. Install a rod that is bolted to the wall.

- Install handrails on each side of the toilet and a raised toilet seat.

- Install grab bars in the shower and/or tub.

- Make sure that the water temperature is set at a safe setting (120 degrees or lower); many older people lose their sensitivity to temperature and can scald themselves.

- Check that the faucets are clearly marked hot and cold. Consider color-coding them with hot being red and blue being cold.

- Organize the medicine cabinet, perhaps color-code the back of the shelves so that cold medicines, prescriptions, and first aid supplies are easily identified.

- Safely position small appliances away from the sink or tub and erect shelving specifically for this purpose.

- Attach a liquid soap dispenser to the wall in the shower so that Mom won't slip and fall when she tries to retrieve a bar of soap she's dropped.

Don't Trip Up on Carpeting

Go through Mom's house, identifying any areas in the carpet that can cause her to trip, and repair them immediately. This is something you should always be on the lookout for during any visit. Having the rug pulled right from under you is never any fun, especially when it's literal. Here are some tips:

- Throw rugs are downright hazardous. Unless we're talking some great family heirlooms, they need to go. (And if it's an heirloom, it might look great on the wall!) Even with carpet tape and no-skid carpet mats, it's easy for a person who scuffles across the floor to slip a shoe under the carpet and trip. It also throws off depth perception because Mom has to readjust her focus back and forth from a bare floor to carpet.

- All stairways should have handrails on both sides.

- Place brightly colored adhesive tape on the edge of each step, so Mom can see the contrast and know she's at the edge of the step.

- If the carpeting on the stairs is loose enough to slip on, it's best to get rid of it altogether.

General Lighting Concerns

Older eyes need more light, pure and simple. They also need the light to be evenly distributed because it takes more time for older eyes to readjust to changing light.

It's similar to how you take a few minutes to adjust from coming inside on a bright sunny day without your sunglasses. Here are some things you can do to accommodate your parent's failing eyesight:

- Dark hallways have got to go, especially, if they lead to brightly lit rooms or a stairway. The lighting should also be indirect, aimed at the ceiling or a wall to prevent glare.

- Install light switches at the top and bottom of stairs. It might be easier for Mom to use those switches that you press rather than flip. It's easier to press with your hand than to use arthritic fingers to flip a tiny switch. You can also install with on/off switches that are lit.

- Arrange for emergency lighting to automatically come on during a power outage.

- Place a flashlight within easy reach on Mom's nightstand. Check on the batteries every few months.

- Install sound or movement activated lights that go on and off automatically when Mom gets up in the night to go to the bathroom.

- For lamps on the nightstand, install adapters that make the lamp go on and off with a mere touch of the hand on the base. (Grandma can show the grandkids her magical powers!)

- Distribute nightlights throughout hallways on route to where Mom might need to go during the night (the bathroom or kitchen, for example). No clutter or cute little tables in the hallways!

- Make sure Mom isn't using extension cords throughout the house where she can trip on them.

One-Floor Living

The last time I thought stairs were fun is when I was a little kid and slid down them when they were newly carpeted. But when I had little kids of my own, terror struck. Those stairs are just as dangerous for your mom. So take a look around the house and see if there is any way to do some innovative redesigning so she's living on one floor.

As I visited families who were taking care of their parents in their two-story homes, I found many a dining room that had become a bedroom. There are two advantages: no more steps up and down to the bedroom, and their parent could feel that they were part of daily life by not being isolated upstairs.

Of course, the dining room alternative works only if you have a bathroom on the same floor. Many older, two-story homes don't have a bathroom on the first floor because it was considered in bad taste. So take a look at closets and see if a bathroom

127

can be installed. It's definitely worth the investment if you can afford it, and it increases the value of the home.

If you can't create a one-floor living arrangement, look into purchasing a stair lift in which your parent sits on a chair that slides up a rail to the top of the steps. There are several companies that sell stair lifts. To find them, look in the Yellow Pages under Medical Equipment, search the Internet using the keywords "stair lifts," or call the National Rehabilitation Information Center at 1-800-346-2742. There are also a number of new Web sites that sell used medical equipment. One such site is www.pemed.com.

If your mom is being discharged from a hospital, ask the social worker if an occupational therapist can be ordered for a site visit to her home. In this instance, Medicare or her HMO may cover the cost of the site visit (be sure to check). The occupational therapist has x-ray vision; she'll see danger spots you and I aren't going to pick up. Make sure you're there to learn what you'll need to do to make Mom's home worthy of the title "There's No Place Like Home."

Sage Source

Call your local area agency on aging (see Appendix B, "National List of State Units on Aging") to see if there are programs available to help you with the costs of renovating the home or give you a low interest loan to do so. You can also contact the Eldercare Locator at 1-800-677-1116.

Sage Source

The American Association of Retired Persons (AARP), along with the Home Builders Association, has a great Web site that gives you ideas and resources on how to design a senior-friendly home for independent living. AARP will also send you a free packet on how to safely remain at home. You can mail a request to AARP Fulfillment EEO#1397, 601 E Street NW, Washington, DC 20049; or order online at www.aarp.org/programs/connect. You can also visit their Web site on home designs at www.aarp.org/universalhome.

Senior-Friendly Lifestyles

Whenever I put off doing some chore as a kid, my mom would say, "What do you think you're doing, living the life of Riley?" I didn't know who Riley was, but if meant taking it easy, I knew it was a good life. So how do we give your parents the "life of Riley"? Remember, this is about offering them a catered lifestyle to make performing the daily tasks of life easier. It isn't about focusing on disabilities or making them feel like they're losing control.

Catered Meals

You might not need this service right away, but if you begin to notice either one of your parents not feeling like preparing food, losing weight, or losing his or her appetite, consider calling the area agency on aging or a local senior center for the nearest Meals on Wheels program in your parents' area. If you sign up with Meals on Wheels, you'll be asked to pay a very modest amount based on your parents' income. Meals on Wheels volunteers can prepare meals for special diets, and for those of you in cold climates, they can also provide "blizzard boxes," which are frozen meals meant to be eaten when volunteers can't get to clients during winter storms.

If you or your siblings enjoy cooking, prepare meals for the week that can easily be popped into the microwave. New services are cropping up every day that will deliver catered meals to the home. (No, not my teenager's version of Meals on Wheels: Pizza Hut.)

Also encourage your parents to get out and join a local senior center where they can eat lunch daily for a small donation for the meal. There are tremendous resources at a senior center besides lunch. It's a great chance for Mom or Dad to get involved in other activities, volunteer, and receive the latest information on health care, healthy living, consumer protection, and insurance. Many senior centers even offer primary health care clinics and exercise programs on site.

Silver Lining

If you, your siblings, and other relatives can't think of what to give your parents for holidays and birthdays, consider buying some personal services such as lawn care, snow removal, and housekeeping. You could also contract with a chore service agency who can come over to fix lights, appliances, doors, locks, or whatever your parents need to have done.

Pills on Delivery and Daily Dispensers

If your mom needs to have her prescriptions filled or refilled, check into local pharmacies that will make home deliveries so she can keep up with her medicines. If Mom is taking quite a few pills, be sure to get her one of those pill organizers you can buy at the pharmacy. Many of these clearly marked plastic organizers can be used for a week's supply of pills that she can organize into as many as four dosages a day—morning, noon, evening, and bedtime. If she is taking a large number of pills, like a friend of mine who has had a kidney transplant, you could get a pill organizer for every day of the week. If you visit your mom weekly, you or a neighbor could fill all the daily organizers for the whole week and avoid any confusion your mom might experience sorting out all those tiny pills. If she has her pills categorized in an organizer, it's easy to know at the end of the day if she's taken all of them. See Chapter 8, "Pills and Your Parents," for details on taking medications.

Sage Source

For easy-to-wear clothing, contact J.C. Penney's catalog department at 1-800-222-6161, AdaptAbility at 1-800-243-9232, or Caring Concepts at 1-800-462-3456. Search on the Web using "easy-to-wear clothing" and "elderly" as your keywords. For products to help out with everyday living, try Independence Living Aids at 1-800-537-2118 or the Access Foundation at 516-568-2715.

Easy Fashions

Buttons and hard-to-reach zippers in the back of dresses are troublesome on arthritic hands. With some creative shopping and a little tailoring, you can make getting "all dolled up" a lot easier. Look for dresses that have zippers with large pulls, shoes with Velcro closures or slip-on shoes, zipperless fashions like dresses that slip over the head with a wide necks, coat-like dresses, wrap-around skirts, or skirts with elastic that just pull up. Get your dad clip-on ties and your mom easy-to-use scarf ties (napkin rings work well). For more casual wear, place elastic shoe strings on sneakers so they slip on while still tied, and don't forget about sweatpants or other pull-on slacks!

No More Bad Hair Days!

My hairdresser volunteers at a nursing home and she has an older clientele. When she heard that I was doing this book she urged me to remind baby boomers how much their mothers love getting their hair done. For many, it is the highlight of the week and it definitely is a mental health boost. So here's another great gift that Mom can't get enough of: gift certificates to her favorite hair stylist. Oh, and don't forget the manicure, a treat you can give her anytime she or the both of you go to the mall.

Gadgets Galore

Thanks to inventive entrepreneurs who've focused on the needs of senior living, there are all kinds of gadgets out there that can make your parents' lives easier. The durable medical equipment (DME) business that I mentioned in the previous chapter is very familiar with what Medicare covers and does not. Almost all of these businesses will deliver what you need and even install it. Just make sure that your mom really needs it. Even though Medicare might cover it, remember, we all are paying for it through our taxes and we need to conserve the Medicare Trust Fund for all of us. It's not free. Some of the things these companies sell—like an egg crate foam mattress—can be picked up at any discount bedding store for a fraction of what DMEs charge. To find a DME near you, just look in the yellow pages under Medical Equipment or Home Health Care.

Can We Talk?

Your mom might not be Joan Rivers, but I'm sure she loves to talk. There are some great phones available today that have large dials, large caller ID displays (something most older people really like and need to identify all of the scam artists trying to sell them something), and accelerated volume in the receiver. You'll need to send over your teenager to program the memory dials and get things set up but it will make Mom's life easier. It's also nice for Mom to have a portable phone that she can take with her when she's in the bathroom so that if she should slip and fall, she can reach someone.

A Real-Life Story

Ironically and sadly, my stepfather died while I was writing this chapter. My mom, who would now live alone, is losing sight in one eye due to macular degeneration. To end this chapter, I'd like to share with you some of the things we did as a family to make living at home easier and safer for my mom. Maybe it will give you some ideas for your own situation:

- Got rid of three throw rugs in the hallways.
- Bought her new hot pads (she was using towels).
- Got her a new phone with big button dials and a built-in caller ID that was easy to read. She's also going to keep the phone number in her husband's name so if someone she calls has caller ID, they won't think she lives alone.
- Bought her a new Rolodex (Mom's real active). We used large font type to print her a new set of name and address cards that she could read more easily.
- Bought her a new calculator with large print.
- Met several of her neighbors and the parish priest, and exchanged phone numbers in case we should need to contact them.
- Since Mom lives 3,000 miles away from all of her four children, we are now co-ordinating our schedules with visits so that one of us or our grown children will be visiting with her every few months.

The Least You Need to Know

- With some modifications to their home, it is possible for your parents to live alone safely and independently.

- Motion-sensitive lighting, lights on timers, security systems, and other ideas can make the outside of a home safer.

- There are hundreds of ways to make Mom's living space senior-friendly; one idea is to get her a personal medical alert system.

- Kitchens and bathrooms are two of the most dangerous rooms in the house for seniors, so be sure to invest the time and money into making them safe.

- There are plenty of community services available to help your parent live alone. Call the Eldercare Locator at 1-800-677-1116 to find out who provides what services.

Chapter 12

Living in the Community: Services and Transportation

In This Chapter

- Tapping into the dozens of community services available for seniors
- Taking advantage of marketing discounts for seniors
- How comfortable does your parent feel driving? A quiz
- Identifying your parents' driving problems and how to prevent and fix them
- Strategies on getting Mom or Dad to retire from driving

With the aging of the American population there has been a near avalanche of community services for older people. It began with a federal law known as the Older Americans Act, passed nearly 30 years ago. This Act gave birth to a myriad of community services for older people, which is often referred to as the "aging network." You'd be surprised at the number of community resources available to your parents, and how many are free. It might take some calling around but it's definitely worth the effort. So before you go off trying to hire help or think that the only way out is to have your parents move into a segregated community or nursing home, take a look at what's out there.

Once you and your parents have found these services, there's the issue of *getting to* them. Ever try telling your dad maybe he should think about giving up the keys to the car? Not a pleasant scene. Retiring from driving is up there with divorce on the stress charts. It is, after all, a divorce of sorts from one of America's greatest love affairs—the car. So how do you know it's time to stop driving? Can your parents safely drive in their 80s? Is public transportation a viable alternative? Read on for some advice.

Services in the Community: First Stop, the AAA

No, I'm not talking about the American Automobile Association. There's another "triple A" out there, and it stands for the area agency on aging. There's one close to you and it's responsible for organizing a wide range of services for your parents in the community. Every county throughout the nation is covered by an area agency on aging. It receives state, federal, and local funds to either set up services or distribute the money to other organizations that offer aging services. Think of the agency as the central hub for all aging services. So, if you want to know what services are available for mom and dad and if your parents are eligible, contacting the aging network's nerve center (area agencies on aging) will save you a lot of time.

Sage Source

You can find your area agency on aging in the phone book listed in the white pages under Area Agency on Aging, or in the government blue pages under Aging or Senior Services. Or call the Eldercare Locator at 1-800-677-1116 for the name and number of the area agency on aging closest to you. You can also contact your state's unit on aging listed in Appendix B, "National List of State Units on Aging." If you're interested in more information on area agencies on aging and what they offer, check out their national association Web site at www.n4a.org.

The area agency on aging is also the major planner for aging services in the community, so it has a good sense of what the needs are among the elderly. This is the agency that also runs the federal Long-term Care Ombudsman Program assigned to every nursing home in the community. The *ombudsman* helps settle conflicts between residents, families, and staff; he or she also reports suspected abuse or neglect and can provide you with very good information regarding quality of care in nursing homes. Every nursing home must post the name and phone number of the ombudsman assigned to it on a bulletin board. You can also track down the ombudsman by calling the area agency on aging listed in your phone book.

Many area agencies on aging distribute funds to senior centers for more local, neighborhood-based services. They also employ teams of professionals who assess whether your parent needs nursing home care or assisted living, and they oversee the elder abuse prevention programs in your community.

All of the area agencies on aging offer information and referral services, so feel free to call upon them to steer you in the right direction.

Geri-Fact

Ombudsman is a Swedish term meaning "representative." The ombudsman's job is to help solve problems between residents, their families, and the staff in long-term care facilities. Every nursing home is assigned an ombudsman, who is usually an employee of the local the area agency on aging.

Senior Centers—More Than Bingo!

Many people think of senior centers as arts and crafts centers where you get a free lunch and top the day off with bingo. If that's what you think, you're definitely behind the times. The senior center of today bustles with a great network of services: health screenings, lunches, consumer information on health care and insurance, primary care clinics, assistance with insurance and paper work, nutrition and healthy lifestyle classes, exercise programs, recreational events, transportation services, volunteer opportunities, computer classes, free e-mail accounts and computer access, and some even offer on-site adult day care.

Every center is different; some will have more activities than others but they are definitely worth a visit to find what connects with your parent. Your parents will make friends and have access to services that will keep them healthy and young—much more so than staying at home on the sofa. Senior centers are listed in your phone book under senior centers or in the blue pages under aging or senior services. The local area agency on aging will have numbers for all of the local senior centers.

Government Agencies

Government agencies at local, state, and federal levels have spent a great deal of attention toward helping families help themselves and protecting older people from scam artists and others who prey on the elderly. Here's my pick of government agencies that can make life better for your mom and dad:

- Local health agencies offer free screenings, flu shots, and information on the quality of local nursing homes. In some states they also oversee personal care homes and home health agencies.

135

- Local housing authorities can tell you about subsidized housing available for low income, older people.

- Local county and city governments often run a parks and recreation program that may include senior centers, field trips, and recreational events. County and city governments also run the transportation system, many of which offer discounts and shared-ride transit services for senior citizens.

- The local county board of assistance as part of the state welfare agency can help you with Medicaid eligibility for nursing home care and other social services that your state offers for low-income seniors.

- The Social Security Office offers a wealth of advice and can process eligibility papers for you. If you don't have a local office near you, visit its Web site at www.ssa.gov or call 1-800-772-1213.

- You may be fortunate enough to live in a community that has a Veterans Administration medical center or an outpatient primary care clinic. To find out, call 1-800-827-1000.

The Phone Book—Go for the Color

Your phone book's blue pages and Yellow Pages offer two excellent ways for you to track down services and resources for your parents. The blue pages list government agencies at the local, state, and federal levels. The listings often explain the kinds of services the agency offers. Many of the listings now include Web site addresses of the agencies. The Yellow Pages—an old standby—is a solid base from which to identify the kinds of services you may need by subject, such as home health care agencies, nursing homes, durable medical equipment, social services, vision services—you name it.

Geri-Fact

Don't forget to look at the beginning of the phone book for lists of emergency services and hotlines.

Another resource is the local United Way agency listed in the white pages. United Way can send you a great directory of community services. And if you live a long distance from your parents, next time you visit grab a local phone book to take back. That way you can make some calls if your mom or dad can't.

Senior Marketing Discounts and Services

Lots of community businesses and hospitals target their services to older consumers. One of the ways to attract them is to offer free services and promotional discounts. So be on the look out for …

- Pharmacies that will make free deliveries.

- Hospitals that offer free screenings, shots, and educational programs, and shuttle services.

- Phone and utility companies that help with bill paying, offer discounts and gadgets to make hearing and seeing easier with a phone, and provide subsidies during the winter for heat and during the summer for air conditioning.

- Grocery stores that make home deliveries; some discount their delivery charges for the homebound. You'll see a lot more of this with the use of the Internet for placing orders.

- Pet services offering discounts that include coming to your mom and dad's home to groom, walk, or get Rover to the vet.

It never hurts to ask just about any business in the service industry whether or not it offers senior discounts. What's to lose?

A Quick Look at Community Services

Kind of Service	What It Is	Where to Find It
Information and referral	Helps you identify what you need and where to get help	Senior centers; area agency on aging; hospitals
Meals on Wheels	Meals delivered to the home for homebound elderly	Senior centers; churches; synagogues; area agency on aging; National Meals on Wheels Foundation (1-800-999-6262)
Telephone reassurance	Volunteers make daily calls to see if everything is okay	Senior centers; area agency on aging
Transportation services	Shared rides (vans) to senior centers, doctors, malls, clinics	Senior centers; public transit authority; area agency on aging
Family caregiver support programs	Services that help families keep older members at home	Senior centers; area agency on aging
Chore services, homemaker	Minor repairs to the home, Mr. Fix-It type services, assistance with household tasks	Senior centers; area agency on aging
Respite care	Care for frail, older people so that family caregivers can take a break	Adult day care centers; nursing homes (some offer care while families go on vacation); area agency on aging

continues

A Quick Look at Community Services   *continued*

Kind of Service	What It Is	Where to Find It
Friendly visitor or companion programs	Volunteer who comes by weekly to visit, run errands; or paid companions to do the same	Senior centers; churches; synagogues; Corporation for National Service (1-800-424-8867)
Adult day care services	Supervised all-day social and recreational programs for people with physical and mental limitations (many have dementia)	Listed in the phone book under Adult Day Care; area agency on aging
Case management, client assessments	Caseworker plans for and arranges services for your parent, and assesses physical and mental functioning	Area agency on aging; Geriatric Care Managers (a private sector company: www.caremanager.com)
Home health care	Range of nursing and nurse's aide care delivered in the home	Listed in the Yellow Pages under Home Health Care Agencies; Visiting Nurses Association
Senior centers	Centers offer meals, social, recreational, and educational activities, health screenings, information, and referral	Listed in the phone book under Senior Centers; area agency on aging; Eldercare Locator (1-800-677-1116)
Employment	Recruit, advise, and assist older workers in finding jobs, re-training programs (for all ages)	Area agency on aging; one-stop job centers (Department of Labor & Industry; blue pages in the phone book)
Legal services, elder protective services, ombudsmen complaint services	Help with financial and legal problems	Area agency on aging; Legal Services, Inc. (blue pages); ombudsman; AARP Legal Hotline (1-800-772-1213)

Getting Around in the Community

Having community services available is one thing, but getting to them is another. The ability to get up and go whenever you please to wherever you please is deep in the American psyche. Where would we be without cars? Having a set of wheels gets Mom and Dad to friends, family, shopping, a job, vacation, the movies, their favorite restaurant, church, golf, bowling, doctor appointments, rehab, volunteering, and educational events. Take the wheels away and they're cut off from the outside world they've created.

If your parents need any of the community services I've been describing to you, then it's likely that they're struggling with conditions that place their ability to drive at risk. For example, if your dad can't do chores anymore because of poor eyesight and he's too shaky on a stepladder; he's probably having trouble yielding the right of way or merging into traffic. If Mom or Dad needs adult day care, he or she definitely shouldn't be driving.

So, how do you know when it's time for your parents to retire from driving? And when they do stop driving, how do you keep them mobile in a car-dependent society?

Senior Alert

According to AARP, the six most common problems with older drivers are failure to yield the right of way, making improper left turns, negotiating blind spots, getting on and off freeways, backing up, and slow reaction times.

Should Miss Daisy Be Driving?

We all age differently and though it's certain that we will have some deficiencies as we age, some of us fare better than others. So assuming that everyone over a certain age should simply stop driving is an unfair assumption and would surely cause a revolution. On the other hand, folks over 80 are more likely than people in any other age group to experience conditions that do affect their ability to drive safely. Vision, especially is affected. The older eye experiences …

- Sensitivity to bright lights causing older drivers to see glare from oncoming traffic at night and on sunny days.

- A decrease in depth perception making parallel parking and left turns very difficult.

- A decrease in the ability to focus resulting in hampered judgment of distances and speed.

- A decrease in peripheral (side) vision leading to difficulties in yielding the right of way.

- Conditions of cataracts (clouding of the lens), glaucoma (squeezed optic nerve) and macular degeneration (blocked central field of vision), which all seriously compromise one's ability to drive.

Besides vision problems, your mom is more likely to experience lack of flexibility in turning her neck when she's backing up or glancing to the side when she's merging into traffic.

Senior Alert

Of all the age groups in the U.S. population, older folks take the most medication. Many of these medications can cause side effects that impair driving. Painkillers, high blood pressure medicines, not eating properly with medications, or not keeping up with fluids can cause confusion and impaired vision and judgment. Make sure your parent is aware of the side effects of medicines—they can be just as lethal a mix as drinking and driving!

Assessing the Situation

One way to assess whether or not any of these conditions or problems are seriously affecting your parents' ability to drive is to have them take you for a spin. Now I suggest you don't whip out a clipboard and test them like your high school driver's ed instructor, but do keep in mind the six most common problems older drivers have (see the earlier Senior Alert sidebar).

If Mom or Dad's driving has some moderate difficulties, then suggest some basic tips such as …

- Identify routes to favorite places that don't use freeways, or involve merges or left-hand turns.
- Get glare-reduction sunglasses for nighttime driving.
- Drive with a passenger to assist with right-of-way decisions.
- Increase the distance between Mom or Dad's car and other drivers to compensate for his or her slower reaction times.
- Suggest your parent take a driver refresher course like AARP's 55 ALIVE Mature Driving Program (see the following Sage Source) to reduce the insurance premium.
- If Mom is having difficulty seeing over the dashboard, go to an auto store and get a seat cushion; you can also pick up a device to raise the gas pedal.
- Start getting your parent to be less car dependent so you can ease Mom or Dad's transition into a nondriver lifestyle. Start arranging transportation to Mom and Dad's favorite places, identify shuttle services, and take advantage of free deliveries (from groceries, pharmacies, doctor's offices).
- Have your parents get their eyesight checked and keep up on the side effects of medications they're taking.

- Add small blind-spot mirrors onto side mirrors.

- Get your parents to apply for a graduated license that excludes night-time driving. This might ease their transition into giving up their full license later. Some insurance companies will offer discounts for graduated licenses that might be the carrot to convince your parents to go for it.

Sage Source

AARP offers a 55 ALIVE Mature Driving Program that gives classes to drivers 50 and older to improve their skills and to avoid accidents and traffic violations. It's an eight-hour course for a mere $10 and is open to anyone. Graduates of the course usually receive discounts on their auto insurance! For a class near you call 1-800-772-1213 or visit the AARP Web site at www.AARP.org/55ALIVE.

The AAA Foundation for Traffic Safety (1-800-305-7233) offers some terrific publications that include a guide for families and a self-exam. A self-exam is also offered by the National Safety Council (1-800-621-6244).

Voluntary Restrictions

Many older drivers voluntarily begin restricting their own driving. The first to go is nighttime driving, quickly followed by ventures on the freeways. Your parents may also decide to stay clear of rush hour and drive only on familiar routes. This might suit them fine, posing few risks to themselves or others. But there will come a time when it is no longer safe for them to be behind the wheel. Like it or not, it's your duty to intervene. If you have doubts about your parent's ability to drive safely, ask Mom or Dad to take the following quiz.

Time to Intervene

Most older people will tell you that they mean to stop driving "someday." They'll go on to say that they'll "face it when they have to," or they'll know when they have to stop. But time slips by and denial sets in and before you know it, they're on the road endangering themselves and every driver along with their precious cargo. You know you have to do something but you, too, have been in denial because the confrontation is just too difficult.

Don't use terms like "giving up the keys," or "you've got to quit driving." Instead start the conversation with "You know, Dad, when you planned your *retirement* from your job, you had a number of things lined up; now that you're approaching *retirement* from driving, what should we line up so that you can get to where you want to go?"

Close Call Quiz: 10 Questions to Ask Yourself
(from AARP's 55 ALIVE Mature Driving Program)

Every day it seems traffic gets more congested, cars move faster, and for many, driving becomes very stressful and, quite simply, a hassle. Is that the case with you?

Ask yourself the following questions.

1. Do you sometimes say, "Whew, that was close"?   ❑ Yes   ❑ No
2. At times, do cars seem to appear from nowhere?   ❑ Yes   ❑ No
3. At intersections, do cars sometimes proceed when you felt you had the right of way?   ❑ Yes   ❑ No
4. Are gaps in traffic harder to judge?   ❑ Yes   ❑ No
5. Do others honk at you?   ❑ Yes   ❑ No
6. After driving, do you feel physically exhausted?   ❑ Yes   ❑ No
7. Do you think you are slower than you used to be in reacting to dangerous driving situations?   ❑ Yes   ❑ No
8. Have you had an increased number of near-accidents in the past year?   ❑ Yes   ❑ No
9. Do you find it difficult to decide when to join traffic on a busy interstate highway?   ❑ Yes   ❑ No
10. Do intersections bother you because there is so much to watch for in all directions?   ❑ Yes   ❑ No

If you answered Yes to any of these questions, you have perhaps had a close call for an accident. It is important to replay and analyze these near-misses because we can learn from them. Ask yourself the following questions:

- Could I have prevented the situation?
- Should I have reacted differently?
- Did I fail to see something?
- Why was the other driver honking at me?

The focus changes from giving up something to continuing to get the same thing but in a different way. By focusing on the word retirement you're tapping into something that most people and society see as positive—an earned rite of passage. If you can line up drivers and other sources of transportation to make life easier, it could be seen as something Dad has earned. This also takes attention away from his disabilities and any hitting on his male ego because he can no longer drive. Let's face it, guys and cars have a special bond we women don't totally get. Plenty of ego is tied up under that hood.

Okay, if you've tried all the approaches and older driver strategies we've gone over and Dad's still putting the pedal to the metal and you won't even get in the car with him, try these:

- Call the Department of Motor Vehicles and ask what your state laws are regarding older drivers. Do they require re-testing of drivers when they reach a certain age? Could they move it up on your dad or mom? Do they have a process for anonymous reporting of unsafe drivers? What happens if you were to report your dad? If he were to be seen by his eye doctor, would the doctor be forced to report his condition (many states have such laws). If all else fails, you may have to report him.

- Convince Dad that if he wants to keep his license then he should see his eye doctor; perhaps new glasses would make the difference. Do let the doctor know of your concerns prior to the appointment and that you want this held in strictest of confidence (unless you're able to bring this up in front of Dad). Let the doctor examine him and decide if he can no longer drive. Most doctors don't like being faced with this issue either, especially if the doctor's been seeing your dad or mom for a good number of years. The doctor may have someone else in the practice see him.

- Try reasoning with your dad by tapping his protective instincts; he's always protected you from harm and would never intentionally hurt anybody. If he keeps driving, he'll hurt some other father's family. You love him a great deal but you've reached a point where you won't place your own kids in the car with him. Appeal to his love of his grandkids. Just focusing on him hurting himself probably won't work—he's still thinking he's invincible.

Geri-Fact

Although drivers over the age of 55 do better than very young drivers, they don't fare as well as drivers age 35 to 54. Drivers age 75 or older are three times more likely to die in a crash than 20-year-old drivers. By 2030, the number of traffic fatalities involving the elderly will be 35 percent greater than the total number of alcohol-related traffic fatalities in 1995.

If all of these strategies fail and you know in your heart that he absolutely should not be driving, it's your civic duty to report Dad to the proper authorities to take his license away. Hiding keys or disengaging the motor won't cut it.

The bottom line? Driving is not a right, it's a privilege. You can't irresponsibly look the other way and hope nothing happens. On the other hand, losing your license can be devastating. For many older people, it marks the beginning of the end. No more independence. Depending upon family and friends on *their* schedules is far too humbling for your independence-loving Dad. Many older folks choose isolation in their home rather than ask for a ride. Giving up the keys solves one problem but it begins a whole host of others if you don't find ways to keep your Dad connected to the community.

Using Public Transportation

Our country has become so car-dependent that our public transportation system has suffered because of it. If you've spent any time in Europe you know what I mean; there are plenty of trains, they're fast, clean, and on time; you even find lots of buses and subways where you're treated to classical music. With the great numbers of older drivers hitting the highways and the onslaught of baby boomers joining their ranks, we better start thinking fast and create a transportation system that is senior friendly.

But in the meantime, who offers what? Many communities offer some sort of shared-ride program where vans pick up older people who cannot use public transportation. They'll take them to doctor's appointments, grocery shopping, malls, and senior centers for a small fee. Call your local transportation authority to find out what's available. If your parent lives in subsidized "Section 8" housing operated by HUD (Housing and Urban Development) the housing development often runs its own van service. Local senior centers also make arrangements with shared-ride programs and cab companies, or run their own vans to pick up seniors who can't get there on public transit. Assisted living centers often offer transportation as part of their package so the elderly can give up their cars when they come to live there. Churches and synagogues often have their own vans that can be used to transport their elder members to grocery stores, services, and special events. Two trips that you could reduce are to the grocery store and to the pharmacy, because many of them now deliver. But don't go overboard on the home delivery route; it's better if Mom and Dad can be out and about, if possible.

Silver Lining

How about getting your parents a driver or using a cab service? You'd be surprised how inexpensive this option can look when you add up the costs of maintaining a car: the gas, inspections, maintenance, and repair, along with the insurance. Break down those monthly costs into how many rides your mom or dad can afford—it's a lot more than you think!

If your parents are retired drivers, take the time to get on the phone and hunt down transportation options for them so they stay active. You'll be doing more for your parents' mental health than any pill ever could.

The Least You Need to Know

- There are a great number of community services available to your parent as part of the "aging network."

- The best place to find out what's available for Mom and Dad is to call your local area agency on aging.

- Older drivers face problems merging, judging distances, and negotiating right-of-way decisions, so help them find alternative routes and get your parents to take driver refresher courses.

- Driving is a privilege. If you won't place your own children in the car with Mom or Dad at the wheel, it's time to do something.

Housing Options

Most older people seem to think that where they live is an all or nothing affair: stay at home or be sent off to a nursing home. With these being the only two choices looming before them, many older folks hold on to their homes for dear life. They do this even if it means they're a prisoner in their own homes—not able to get out while remaining isolated in neighborhoods they no longer recognize. To the contrary, there are quite a few options out there for a creative alternative to living *home alone*.

All of these options assume that your parents are in basically good health and can live independently. If they need a moderate amount of assistance in the tasks of everyday living and it's not safe for them to live alone, consider assisted living, which I discuss in Chapter 14, "Assisted Living."

Senior Apartments

Most communities have at least one apartment complex that is dedicated to renting solely to seniors. Many of these have been constructed and are maintained by the federal Department of Housing and Urban Development (HUD). If the senior apartment is operated by HUD, then the residents are low income and receive subsidized rent from the government. You'll need to check with your local housing authority to determine eligibility limits for your parents because limits vary from state to state. This type of high-rise is usually referred to as Section 202 housing in reference to the section of the law that authorized HUD to build these in the first place.

These apartments have been built with seniors in mind, offering them handicapped-accessible rooms and transportation services, and many offer congregate meals in a dining hall within the building. Community agencies often offer services on-site and have a referral relationship with the agency that runs the facility. Local housing authorities are eligible to compete for funds that offer recreational and social services to those living in these facilities. So, depending upon how active your local housing authority is, you might find a lot of activities being offered at the high-rise. Many times the housing development also has a strong relationship with a local senior center, or a center can actually operate out of the high-rise.

This type of living option offers your mom or dad the chance to socialize with others, receive services, and maintain privacy and independence at a modest cost.

With a growing Baby Boomer market in sight, the private sector is busy building apartment complexes or refurbishing older ones designed for senior-friendly living. Many of the ground floors have convenience stores with banking services, security guards, transportation services, and handicapped-accessible rooms. There is quite a price range for these apartments, and, of course, it depends upon what services and features your mom or dad wants.

Sage Source

HUD operates a special Web site (www.hud.gov/senior) for seniors regarding housing issues. HUD also offers housing counseling centers. Call HUD at 1-888-569-4287 to find the center nearest you.

Geri-Fact

There is usually a waiting list to get into Section 202 apartments. I've known some friends who have waited two years or more. Call the area agency on aging (1-800-677-1116) to find the Section 202 housing nearest your parents or call the local housing authority in the blue pages of your phone book. If your parents want to eventually move into the high-rise, get on the list now.

Real estate agencies often have special agents who can help you search for these apartment complexes. A real estate agent might also be aware of a complex that may have a decidedly older clientele yet it is basically intergenerational—something that your parent might enjoy.

College Days Are Here Again: House Mates

Why live in a big old house alone? Seniors, especially older women who survive their husbands, are finding that it makes a lot more sense to share a house along with the expenses rather than relocate. They can share food expenses, utilities, and pool their resources to maintain the home and split up tasks between each other. Kind of like Mary Tyler Moore and Rhoda, but in the same house. The trick here is finding someone your mom is compatible with and then deciding whose house she lives in— hers or her friend's?

If she doesn't have a friend in mind then you can place an ad in the paper and interview and research the applicant's references. Or she could find someone through a local faith-based organization or senior center.

Besides the technicalities in a lease agreement, your mom needs to think through what she and her roommate expect of each other: Do they share chores and which ones; do they share meals; what about smoking and sharing mutual space like the living room and kitchen; what about visitors, pets, and the laundry? If they want to maintain their friendship or establish one, these questions should be openly discussed and decided upon before the questions pop up in daily life.

Senior Alert

If your mom takes in more than two unrelated roommates, make sure she's checked with the zoning board. She could be treading close to running a boarding home or owning multifamily housing, which might be prohibited in her neighborhood. Your mom sure isn't looking to be on the wrong side of the law!

Sage Source

The National Resource Center on Supportive Housing and Home Modification provides excellent information on how to modify the home, resources available to finance modification, and supportive services to help your parent stay at home. The Center is run by the Andrus Gerontology Center at the University of Southern California. Visit www.homemods.org, or call at 213-740-1364.

Accessory Apartments

In keeping with our roommate theme, single-family homes with enough space can be converted into a separate accessory apartment, which your mom or dad can rent out.

Converting surplus space into an accessory apartment can give older homeowners additional income, companionship, security, and the opportunity to trade services for rent (transportation for home maintenance, for example). On the other hand, if your parent wants to become a tenant, this option offers affordable rent for older people who no longer need their large homes or the hassles of home ownership.

If you want to lease out part of your home, you will need to get a building permit and zoning permission to renovate the home for an accessory apartment. Some area agencies on aging have programs to help seniors create accessory apartments, so give them a call.

ECHO Housing

If you have the land and want your parent near, but neither of you wants to live under one roof like the Waltons, then here's a creative solution: It's called Elder Cottage Housing Opportunity (ECHO), a modular home that can temporarily be placed on your property. Don't forget to visit the zoning folks; the fact that the unit is considered temporary makes it more acceptable to many zoning boards.

Silver Lining

If your parent is receiving medical assistance from the state, foster care may be covered under Medicaid. In this instance, you'll know that the foster family has undergone a rigorous review by the state welfare office. Each state has its own regulations on foster care, so it's best to call your local area agency on aging or local welfare office to find out what options are available for your parent.

These modulars are about the size of a garage and are designed for senior living: one floor, a bedroom, kitchen, handicapped-accessible bathroom, and living room. Many of these modulars can be designed to fit the architecture of your home so it doesn't look so out of place. Mom maintains her privacy and independence, and you both gain the security of being there for each other. The average ECHO unit is about $25,000 and about 550 square feet. Manufacturers of mobile homes are a good source to find out who sells these in your community.

Foster Care: It's Not Just for Kids

Though certainly not as commonplace as foster care for children, foster care for older people is becoming popular with more and more families.

Many older folks seek this kind of living arrangement because they do have some limitations in the tasks of daily living. They need the foster family to prepare their meals, transport them, and do the laundry, and they require a watchful eye so they don't wander off or become hurt. This is not a suitable arrangement if your mom or dad requires daily medical supervision or care.

Other families offer their services privately and will take in an older person for a monthly fee. In this instance, be sure to check out references, the home's safety, and its cleanliness. Take your time looking over the contract—know exactly what you are signing. The best assurance of quality is frequent visits on your part or, if you live a long distance away, enlist a family friend or neighbor who can visit frequently and report back to you.

Continuing Care Retirement Communities (CCRCs)

If your mom and dad want it all and can afford it, this is a great housing option. Referred to as CCRCs or life care communities they offer it all on one campus: independent living apartments and homes, assisted living apartments, and nursing home care. A wide variety of activities are offered: golf, swimming, exercise equipment, physical therapy, hairstylists, and educational courses. Their dining halls are usually designed as fine dining restaurants. Transportation services are provided and many field trips are arranged. The community is extremely active. They also have the peace of mind knowing that if they do become ill, they can receive care right on the campus—even nursing home care. It is similar to living in a village of elders. Many also offer overnight housing for families when they come to visit grandma.

This housing option is not provided on a monthly basis like most others. In this instance, your parents will pay an entrance fee anywhere from $25,000 to $300,000, depending on how high-end a place they can afford. In addition, they will pay a monthly fee that can range from $500 to $3,000, depending on what services your parents want.

When it comes to researching this type of facility there are a few things you should do, as outlined in the following sections.

Check Out Their Financial Solvency

Your mom and dad are probably going to invest most of their life savings into this venture, so—besides making sure that the quality is good—you'll want to be guaranteed that the company is financially secure and reputable. Not all states regulate CCRCs; right now the number is at 38, and you have to track down which department in your state government does the regulating. Some states appoint their human services department to oversee CCRCs, while others appoint their health department or insurance commissioner. Check out your state's governmental Web site for more information or call your state's general number to find out which, if any, agency regulates CCRCs. Ask if they'll send you a directory of CCRCs in the state. Another resource is your state's attorney general's office, which can inform you of any litigation or fines that have been issued against the company.

Ask if They Are Accredited by the CCAC

The American Association of Homes and Services for the Aging (AAHSA) sponsors the Continuing Care Accreditation Commission (CCAC), which inspects and accredits CCRCs. You can find out whether the one you're interested in has been accredited by simply asking, or by contacting the CCAC at 202-783-2242 or www.ccaconline.org. At the Web site you can review a list of all CCRCs that have been accredited by the association. Many of them have their own Web sites that you can link to.

Silver Lining

The American Association of Homes and Services for the Aging, which accredits CCRCs, is a trade association; so CCRCs that are accredited have volunteered and paid a fee to be inspected by their own association. Some people feel that this is a conflict of interest and, as a result, some CCRCs with high standards have opted out of the process. Others contend that the standards are stringent and do provide a solid marker of good care from a well respected nonprofit organization. An accreditation by AAHSA is a good quality standard for you to consider.

Three Kinds of Agreements

There are basically three kinds of agreements that CCRCs offer:

1. **Extensive contract.** This contract is all-inclusive offering unlimited long-term nursing care for little or no substantial increase in your parents' usual monthly payments.

2. **Modified contract.** This includes a specified amount of limited long-term nursing home care. Once your parent has used the limit then he or she is responsible for paying the bill in full. Remember Medicare does not cover nursing home care!

3. **Fee-for-service.** No nursing home coverage is offered; your parent is required to pay the bill out-of-pocket or carry long-term care insurance. Independent and assisted living services are covered.

Your parent will need to sign a very detailed contract to become a member of the CCRC. Given the amount of money involved and the complexity of the agreement, it's highly recommended to have both a lawyer and an accountant look over the agreement.

Questions You'll Want to Ask

If you're considering a CCRC, make sure you ask these questions:

- Who makes the decision as to what level of care your parent needs, especially after Mom or Dad has become ill?
- What kind of refund policy does it offer and under what circumstances?
- Are there health insurance requirements (must your parent have certain kinds of coverage)? Does the CCRC purchase long-term care insurance on your parents' behalf? With what company?
- Is the CCRC subject to licensure by any state agency? Which ones? Ask to see the most recent inspection reports.
- What is the payment schedule? Do residents own or rent their apartments?
- Is the CCRC accredited?

House-Rich but Cash-Poor

For most of us, our home is our greatest asset both emotionally and financially. For older people, most of their net worth is usually tied up in their home. The problem is they need to sell it to reap the financial gain of their diligent payments. And that's something many parents don't want to do even when they find themselves financially strapped keeping up with repairs on the house. There are some financing options you and your parents can consider. But watch out: There are a lot of scam artists out there! Be sure to work with a reputable lending institution and do your research.

Reverse Mortgages

You probably haven't thought of your monthly mortgage as a forward mortgage but if you think of it that way you'll get the reverse mortgage concept. In the forward mortgage you pay a lender a monthly payment in anticipation that you'll eventually own the home. With the reverse mortgage, you own your home and the lender pays you a monthly payment in anticipation of eventually owning it as an asset. The lender is betting that the property value will remain the same or appreciate and the lender will be paid from the sale of the house once your parents move or die. Meanwhile, your parents can live on this income, which can help with health care expenses and enhance the quality of their lives. Of course, this option works only if your parents have paid off their mortgage, or most of it.

One of the more popular reverse mortgages, also known as home equity conversion loans, is the tenure loan. This allows homeowners to stay in their homes until they die or move. The payment is calculated based upon your parents' life expectancy, projections on the property's appreciation, interest rate, and property value among other things. Be aware that you must pay closing costs and insurance premiums which can reach up to $10,000. If you parents are on Medicaid or Supplemental Security Income (SSI), they can receive this income as long as they spend it within the month and are not piling it up as an asset. It must be used for living expenses.

Deciding on whether or not a reverse mortgage is the best option for your parents isn't one of those no-brainers. Your parents have to ask themselves: Do I want to spend my equity now? How long do I expect to live? What do I do, if I need nursing home care? Do I mind not leaving my house to my family as part of my estate? How will this improve the quality of my life? What will happen to the value of my house? Will this allow me to live independently? Does this financially yield the best results for me?

Senior Alert

Absolutely know what you're doing when it comes to home equity conversions. You've got to watch out for "equity sharing fees," also known as cost bubbles, which is how companies can get around truth-in-lending disclosures and the wide variance in credit lines. The Web site www.reverse.org gives you very objective information on reverse mortgages. The *Washington Post* calls the site "scrupulously independent … the first step for smart consumers." For more information, contact the National Center for Home Equity Conversion, 360 N. Robert Street, #403, St. Paul, MN 55101.

The Department of Housing and Urban Development (HUD) offers reverse mortgages. Call HUD at 1-888-466-3487 to see if your parents qualify. AARP offers a list of reverse mortgage counselors, a *Home Made Money Guide,* and a 30-minute video called *Reverse Mortgage Choices.* To order, call AARP at 202-434-6042, or visit AARP's Web site at www.aarp.org.

Property Tax Deferral Program

Property taxes for many older people who are living on a fixed income can become a major burden. Some states offer a program in which your parents can defer payments of their home property taxes until they sell their home or die. Usually, this type of deferment is based on income guidelines—it's not for the rich and famous. Call your local taxing body or the area agency on aging to see if this option is offered in your parents' area.

Moving

Hey, this is everybody's favorite. I'm surprised that Martha Stewart hasn't told everyone that the best way to clean house is to simply move every five years!

If the thought of moving paralyzes your parents, especially if Mom or Dad lives alone, there are some new guys in town. A good number of big-name realty companies now have special divisions that are specifically geared to helping older people move. They'll come in and organize a sale of their furniture, help them figure out what to bring to the new living quarters, and make the move—and even help them design their new living space. Call around and find out who offers this service. It saves a lot of headaches.

You can also call on professional organizers found in the Yellow Pages under "Organizing Services" or contact the National Organization of Professional Organizers at 512-206-0151 or visit Web sites at www.napo.net or www.livingtransitions.com. Here are a few tips from organizers: have your parent choose five of the most important pieces of furniture she must have to feel at home in her new place, take photos of furniture that has special meaning, ask your parent to tell you the story behind furniture and artifacts being given away to family members, then write it on a piece of paper and place it inside the item or tape it to the back of it to pass on to future generations. To get parents into the swing of moving—start with items in the basement to give away or sell. Chances are they aren't as emotionally tied to them.

The Least You Need to Know

- Your parent doesn't have to be relegated to living home alone; they can opt for ECHO housing, rent or find accessory apartments, take in a roommate, or look into foster care.

- If your parent qualifies for Section 202 housing and wants to live there, get on the list now!

- CCRCs can give your parents everything they need from independent living through nursing home care—all in one place—if they can afford it.

- Reverse mortgages can present a great opportunity for cash flow, but do your homework first.

- Moving your parents doesn't have to be a headache: Several large realty companies now offer services geared toward helping seniors make the move.

Assisted Living

Probably one of the most confusing things about assisted living is defining it. You'll hear it referred to in a number of ways: catered living, boarding homes, personal care homes, board and care homes, and, finally, assisted living. Whatever they are called, they are somewhere between nursing home care and independent living and they vary widely in what they offer.

The people who live in these facilities do need moderate assistance in the tasks of daily living. So, if your dad has reached a point where it's not safe having him live alone and he is not sick enough to receive nursing home care, then assisted living is an option for him to consider.

Who Shouldn't Go to an Assisted Living Facility?

One way of helping you sort through whether or not an *assisted living facility* would work for your parents is getting to the bottom line right away. So, who *shouldn't* go?

Geri-Fact

Assisted living facilities provide 24-hour coordinated and supervised support in a group residential setting. They offer a wide range of services for seniors that promote independence and privacy while providing a safe, supervised environment. They also provide meals and custodial care such as housekeeping and transportation services.

Most facilities will not take anyone who suffers from moderate to severe dementia or is incontinent unless they operate a special dementia unit and are licensed to do so. Don't try to sneak your parent in by not telling the full truth about any level of dementia. Most facilities are simply not set up to care for people with dementia and multiple health problems. As a result, your parent may fall into harm's way.

If your mom or dad has extensive medical problems that require daily monitoring, but he or she doesn't require nursing home care, you'll need to search for a facility that has the staffing and training to care for you parent. All assisted living facilities are not alike and they do not have to meet the stringent care standards of nursing homes. The care standards vary from state to state.

Who *Should* Go?

The goal of assisted living is to make performing the tasks of daily living easier and safer. Living with other folks has added benefits. People find themselves eating better, exercising, and enjoying newfound friends. The social networks that develop are very strong and can do a great deal for Mom or Dad's outlook on life. Plus, your parent's chances of getting exercise and eating well are significantly increased by living in an environment with a bunch of buddies. With staff around to look out for their well-being, parents often make marked improvements once they've left the isolated, sedentary lifestyle of living alone.

You and your parents also have the security of being near other people and having a 24-hour on-site staff available in case of an emergency. Assisted living makes sense when Mom or Dad is having difficulty in performing the activities of daily living to such an extent that he or she either has a real hard time doing them or can't perform them at all. It's also reached a point where it's simply no longer safe to leave them totally alone.

If they are having moderate to extreme difficulty in performing two or three of the following tasks, assisted living just might be the answer.

Activities of daily living:

- Bathing
- Eating
- Using the toilet
- Grooming
- Dressing

Tasks of everyday life:

- Shopping
- Housekeeping
- Using transportation
- Taking medication
- Reading
- Communicating
- Cooking
- Doing laundry
- Managing money
- Using the phone
- Maintaining a home

The activities of daily living are known as ADLs; the tasks of everyday life are known as instrumental ADLs. So, if you want to impress the geriatricians, tell them how your parents are doing with their ADLs!

You'll find that most of the people who live at these facilities are active and basically in good to fair health. They have, however, health conditions or age-related disabilities that make living alone tough and in some instances unsafe. You'll see people there who will be using walkers and wheelchairs, while others are able to move around on their own. They enjoy the social stimulation of meals at the dining hall and remain fairly active. They prefer a catered lifestyle where they don't have to cook, maintain a home, clean, or do laundry (my teenage son obviously thinks he's living in one).

Chances are the assisted living facility will want your parent to have an examination to determine his or her physical and mental health along with the ability to perform activities of daily living. These facilities are rightfully concerned that they might bring someone in who has needs that are over their heads. If they don't seem worried about this—you should!

What Do Assisted Living Facilities Look Like?

These facilities can range from a house that someone has divided into rooms (boarding house origins) taking in three to 20 people, to a large complex of residencies into the hundreds. For example, a well-known hotel chain is building a great number of these facilities throughout the country that look like colonial southern mansions with large wraparound porches.

Some of the facilities stand alone while others are part of a complex or campus that also offers independent living apartments for people who need no assistance and nursing home care for those who are very sick. Assisted living facilities that are part of this scenario are part of a continuing care retirement community that I told you about in the previous chapter.

What Mom or Dad Should Expect

Assisted living facilities do vary in what they offer but here's the *least* they should offer:

- Three nutritious meals a day
- Housekeeping
- Laundry
- Minimal amount of supervision (checking in on your parent every day to make sure that he or she is okay)
- Some social-recreational activities

- A pleasant, private, clean, furnished room
- A safe environment
- Handicapped-equipped bathroom facilities
- Twenty-four-hour staff on the premises

Silver Lining

Staff take notice of those residents who have family looking in on them, so visit your parent often. Be sure to vary the time of day you visit so that you get to know different staff. If you live out of town, develop a relationship with the staff and call every week. Be sure to let the staff know how much you appreciate them.

Many facilities also offer other services and usually charge for them. Here's some of the things that you may want to arrange for your parents:

- **Assistance with daily medications.** Only a registered nurse who is certified to "pass meds" can actually administer medications to your parent. However, an aide could remind your parent to take his or her medications, and place it out for him or her, but your parent has to take the medication without assistance. You could also request an aide to place your parents' medications in a daily or weekly dispenser.

- **Assistance with bathing.** Nurse's aides have the training to assist your parent with a shower. Make sure that the shower and bathroom facilities have safety bars, a chair for sitting in the shower, no-skid floors, and a call button for help.

- **Assistance with other daily living tasks.** Depending upon your parents' needs and the level of care the personal care home provides, the staff at the facility may also provide partial assistance with dressing, walking, bathing, using the toilet, and eating. (Please note the word *partial*. These facilities are not for people who are totally dependent in these services.) You should also ask if the staff is able to bring meals to your parent's room if Mom or Dad isn't feeling well enough to go to the common dining room.

- **Transportation.** Most facilities provide some type of transportation service to various common sites in the area such as shopping malls, senior centers, and doctor's offices.

Who Regulates Them?

For the most part, assisted living facilities are regulated by government agencies which are similarly involved in licensing a businesses to operate hotels: The construction of the facility has to meet building codes and zoning requirements, the kitchen and dining facilities have to meet the same requirements as does any restaurant, and the building must meet fire and safety codes. Multiple state agencies will be involved, such as the department of agriculture, department of environmental resources, department of health, and department of labor and industry, and so will local government fire and safety authorities. If it is a small facility, say for instance under 20 people, the state inspectors may make exceptions to some of the architectural requirements.

Senior Alert

In most states, assisted living facilities are unregulated. No licenses are given to them to meet certain standards of care like skilled nursing facilities. So you're on your own. You really need to take the time to research the facility to make sure it meets your parents' needs.

Sage Source

Some assisted living facilities are voluntarily going through an accreditation process that was launched in January 2001. These facilities are being reviewed by experts in the field to determine if they meet certain standards. The national group that accredits them is CARF: the Rehabilitation Accreditation Commission. Ask the facility if they have a certificate from CARF or visit their Web site at www.carf.org. You can also search for facilities that are members of the nonprofit group AAHSA (American Association of Homes and Services for the Aging) at their Web site: www.AAHSA.org.

If the facility admits people who are on Medicaid (medical assistance), that state's department of welfare, department of health, or department of human services *may* require the facility to meet certain standards of care and staffing for which the state will issue a license. You'll need to ask the facility if it takes Medicaid. If it does, ask to see a copy of a recent inspection report.

Doing Your Homework

Location and affordability are the first two factors you should consider while searching for a facility. Most people want to be close enough so that relatives and friends can maintain contact. And as with everything else in life, you can buy only what you can afford, so figure out what your parent can afford every month. Most facilities operate on a monthly fee basis.

Once you've zeroed in on a few facilities, you'll need to set up appointments to see the facilities and talk with the administrator of each one. Here's a checklist of what to look for in a facility and what questions to ask. It's a good idea to make a copy to take with you when you visit. Don't leave home without it!

Your Guide to Interviewing and Inspecting an Assisted Living Facility

Is the facility state licensed?
- What kind of license and the date of the license?
- Does it accept Medicaid?

Who owns the facility?
- Is it run by a large corporation or chain?
- Is it a nonprofit or profit organization?
- Is it a religious (faith-based) facility?
- Is it run by individuals?
- Is it affiliated with a nursing home?

Word to the wise: Finding out who is legally responsible and operates the facility helps you track down its record and reputation with the Better Business Bureau and government agencies. Some religious and nonprofit homes will help subsidize payments.

What's the capacity: How many people are allowed to reside in the facility?
- How many residents currently live here?
- On average, how long do residents live here?

Word to the wise: Find a place that is filled close to capacity and where people have been residents for a long period of time.

How many staff are employed full-time?

- Can you describe their positions?
- How many aides do you employ? Are they certified as nursing assistants?
- What's the average length of employment of your employees?
- How many staff are employed part-time?

Word to the wise: Watch out for facilities that have high staff turnover rates, or too few staff to care for a large number of residents. If the residents appear to have quite a few needs, then the facility is probably understaffed.

- What kind of ongoing training does your staff receive?
- Has all your staff been cleared by a background check (police check and state registry for nursing assistants)?
- Could you please describe the needs of the current residents?
- What percentage are wheelchair bound?
- What percentage need help with eating?
- What percentage need help with bathing?

Word to the wise: If these percentages are high, make sure the facility has a good staff-to-resident ratio because these folks are going to need a significant amount of help every day.

What core services does the facility offer under the monthly rate?

1. Meals

- How many a day?
- If my parent is sick, will you deliver to the room?
- Is there a dietician overseeing the menus?
- Can I see a copy of last month's menu?
- Can you meet my parents' special diet needs (for example, healthy heart diet, diabetic diet)?
- Do you provide assistance with eating?
- Who prepares the meals? What is their training?

2. Daily Living Task Assistance

- What kind of housekeeping will be done in my parent's room and how often?
- What laundry services do you provide?

continues

continued

- Does my parent need to bring his or her own linens (washcloths, towels, sheets, pillowcases)?
- How often is the bedding changed?
- Do you wash all clothing or is this an extra charge?
- What personal belongings can my parent bring (such as small appliances like a microwave, humidifier, small refrigerator; bedroom furniture, chairs, wall hangings)?
- Is there a dry cleaning service?
- Do you provide assistance with bathing?
- What kind of training does the person have who assists?
- What kind of safety features are installed in the bathroom?
- Is there an emergency call button in the bathroom?

Is transportation provided?

- Where to?
- Can arrangements be made for doctor's appointments?
- Is there a charge? How much?

Are there any formal relationships with hospitals, primary care clinics, and nursing homes?

- Do you help my parent get help if he or she gets sick?
- Is there a physician on call?
- Should my parent have his or her own physician?
- If my parent is out for an extended period of time such as in the hospital or at a rehab facility, does my parent keep the room and is there a lesser charge?
- Do physical therapists, occupational therapists, and speech therapists come regularly to the facility?
- Will the facility automatically call me if my parent is sick?

What social and recreational activities are offered?

- May I see a copy of the most recent month's activity calendar?
- Are the activities varied and interesting? Do the residents have input in planning the activities?

What safety features does the facility provide?

- Does it have a sprinkler system?
- Are there adequate numbers of smoke detectors?

- Are there handrails in the hallways?
- Are there panic buttons in the rooms?
- Is there air conditioning? (Heat waves are lethal to older people, so make sure there is proper temperature control for all seasons.)
- How does the facility protect older people from wandering off (and yet, not lock them in case of a fire)?
- What is the fire escape plan?
- Is the staff bonded in case of theft?

What extra services are offered and what is the charge? For example:

- Do you provide assistance with finances and bills—taking residents to the bank, help with paying bills, etc.? (Be sure there is no conflict of interest. Chances are, however, that most of your parent's monthly income will be going directly to the assisted living facility. Look into paying bills for your Mom or Dad electronically and having all income directly deposited into his or her account.)
- How much does telephone service cost? What does the facility provide for residents who do not have a private phone? Does each resident have their own line?
- Is there a hairdresser or barber on the premises? What are the rates?
- Is massage therapy available? What is the cost?
- Do you offer dry cleaning pickup and delivery? How often? What is the cost?

Checking Out Their Reputation

Even though many assisted living facilities are *not* licensed, there are many agencies that do come in contact with them because they refer or treat people who are living at the facility. If I were doing some detective work for you on tracking down their reputation, here's who I'd call:

- Your area agency on aging (AAA): They are listed in the yellow pages; ask for the ombudsman's office. Or check Appendix B, "National List of State Units on Aging."
- Local senior center (ask the AAA for the closest one to you, or check out the blue pages in your phone book under Adult Services).
- Local Hospital (ask for their social work department).
- Local Union (such as the Services Employee International Union).
- Local and state department of health.

- Local and state department of welfare.
- Better Business Bureau.
- State attorney general's office (many have a consumer protection office).

What Do They Cost?

The cost of staying at an assisted living facility varies widely; of course, much of the cost depends on the services that are provided. The average monthly rate can range anywhere from $350 to $3,500. Some facilities want one month in advance, others might want a set amount upfront, and others work on a monthly fee basis.

If your mom is low income and is on the state's Medicaid program, she might also be eligible for Supplemental Security Income (SSI). You can use both of these incomes to make a monthly payment to the assisted living facility. *Please note that most states do not reimburse assisted living facilities directly:* They pay your parent and then your parent pays the facility. In contrast, when it comes to nursing homes, the state pays them directly and requires that the nursing home meet certain health and safety requirements at annual inspections.

Some states, however, have special programs to assist people with the expenses of assisted living. Call your local area agency on aging to find out what is offered in your state.

Geri-Fact

Personal care, custodial care, and assisted living are *not* covered by Medicare. If your parent has a long-term care insurance policy, he or she might have paid additionally for this service, but it's unlikely. Most of the assisted living bill in this country is out of pocket. (For more on Medicare, see Chapter 21, "Got to Have Those M&Ms: Medicare and Medicaid.")

The Least You Need to Know

- Most assisted living facilities are not licensed for their quality of care or staff
  by any government agency.
- Narrow your list down to a couple of places based on affordability and location, then do your research.
- Visit the facility and ask all of the questions on our checklist.
- Research the facility's reputation by calling the local ombudsman at the area agency on aging.
- Develop a good relationship with the assisted living staff and visit often.

Chapter 15

Choosing a Nursing Home

In This Chapter

- Who needs nursing home care?

- What Medicare and Medicaid cover—and what they don't

- Other payment options

- Tips on finding a quality nursing home

- The importance of doing your homework

- Read the fine print and know what you're agreeing to

Should your parent go into a nursing home? This is one of the tougher decisions you will ever make, but about one third of the time the decision is made for you due to a medical crisis. A debilitating brain or heart attack, fast progression of dementia, or a hip fracture or another physical condition that is clearly beyond your family's or home health aide's ability to treat makes the decision a little easier. In these instances, you don't have much of a choice.

The decision gets tougher when your parent is sick and dependent, yet with adequate home health care Mom or Dad is able to remain at home. In this instance you must balance your parent's needs and desires along with your family's resources and commitment to keeping Mom or Dad at home. No matter what the circumstance, your mom and dad, if they are able to communicate, must be part of this decision. And if they can't share their thoughts with you, keep their values in mind while you choose a nursing home.

What Is a Nursing Home?

Nursing homes are also called long-term care facilities. They offer skilled nursing care, rehabilitation, medical services, protective supervision, and assistance with the tasks of daily living to people with long-term illnesses. Many of the residents have physical and mental impairments that require living in a fully supervised environment. Nursing homes are staffed with registered nurses, a medical director (physician), and certified nursing assistants. Therapists in such fields as physical therapy, occupational therapy, speech therapy, and music therapy are either employed or contracted by the facility. The facility also offers recreational and social activities for residents.

Geri-Fact

There are 16,800 nursing homes and two thirds of them are part of for-profit chains. Just over 1.6 million people on any given day are being cared for in nursing homes. That's 4 percent of those 65 years and older in the United States.

Nursing homes are inspected and surveyed by state and federal government agencies to maintain their licenses. Both state and federal laws govern the standards that nursing homes must satisfy to stay in business. There's more on what you should know about these laws later in this chapter.

Who Goes to Nursing Homes?

People with long-term mental or physical conditions that require a 24-hour protective environment with medical and health care services need nursing home care. A physician must make the determination of whether or not your mom or dad needs nursing home care. A diagnostic workup must be given to justify your parent needing this level of care. This isn't something that you, your parents, and your siblings just up and decide one day. Nursing homes are for chronically ill and debilitated people. Most of the residents are well up in age; over half of all women over the age of 85 years live in nursing homes while one out of three men that age do.

Here are some of the characteristics of nursing home residents, as reported by the federal Agency for Health Care Policy & Research in 1996:

- Half of all residents have some form of dementia, half have some form of heart disease, and one out of five has suffered a stroke.
- The average age of a nursing home resident is 85 years.
- Just over half of all residents are incontinent (bowel and bladder).
- One in 15 residents is on a ventilator or dialysis, or is receiving some other form of specialized treatment.

- Over 80 percent have great difficulty with three or more activities of daily living such as bathing, dressing, eating, using the toilet, walking, or getting in and out of chairs or bed.

It is also common today to find patients from hospitals being transferred to nursing homes for short stays. Nearly 40 percent of nursing home admissions are for recuperation from surgery or an illness. The reason for the transfer is that it's cheaper for the hospital to transfer your parent to the nursing home to recuperate than to rack up the high cost of a hospital stay.

Geri-Fact

According to the latest figures from the Health Care Financing Administration, as a nation (government, insurance, and you) we spent nearly $360 billion on hospital care in 1996, as opposed to $78 billion on nursing home care. Care in a hospital averages about $1,000 a day. Care in a nursing home is about $1,000 for a whole week. No wonder hospitals and Medicare are transferring people to nursing homes to recover—it's a lot cheaper.

Who Pays?

And you thought college tuition was a budget breaker! How about $45,000 a year for the average nursing home stay? No low-interest student loans or scholarships here. So what's a typical, middle-income family to do? If your parents were fortunate enough and well-off enough to have purchased long-term care insurance then the financial hit will be minimal. But if they don't have it, which accounts for 98 percent of us, here's what you should know.

Medicare

Under very limited conditions Medicare will pay for *some* nursing home care costs for those who require skilled nursing or rehabilitation services. Here's a shocker: Medicare pays for less than *10 percent* of all nursing home bills! Most people think Uncle Sam picks up the tab. Wrong.

If you are fortunate enough to have some of the bill paid by Medicare, then you've got to make sure that your parent goes to a home that is certified by Medicare. Not all are, so make sure you ask. Here are the five conditions your parent must meet before Medicare will pay for any care:

1. Skilled care is required every day as an inpatient.

2. Your parent has been in the hospital for three consecutive days, not including the day of discharge.

3. Admission to the nursing home is made within 30 days of the hospitalization.

4. Admission to the nursing home is for the same condition as was the hospitalization.

5. A physician must certify the need for skilled nursing or rehabilitative care.

If your parent meets all of these conditions Medicare *may* pay up to the first 20 days of your parent's nursing home stay. After the first 20 days Medicare, as of January 2003, will expect you to pay up to $105 per day for days 21-100, so hopefully your parents have a Medi-gap policy to help with the bill. After the 100 days, you're on your own. Please pay attention to the words—*limited, some,* and *may*—there aren't any guarantees. Be sure to ask the hospital social worker to explain the conditions and terms to you.

Bottom line? Don't count on Medicare to pay your parent's nursing home bill!

Medicaid

Medicaid programs are run by the state, usually the department of public welfare or human services. Medicaid pays the nursing home costs for people who have a low income and limited assets. Today, Medicaid pays for seven out of 10 residents—it's why state welfare budgets are hemorrhaging.

Most people start out paying for nursing home care through their own savings and spend down to a point where they qualify for Medicaid. Every state has different rules for qualifying, so you should contact your local area agency on aging or welfare office to find out your state's eligibility requirements.

Sage Source

State Health Insurance Assistance Program (SHIP) offers trained volunteers who can help you sort through your parents' insurance issues, such as figuring out what coverage they currently have, whether or not they qualify for other government programs, or if they have policies that duplicate each other. They can't recommend a specific policy but can answer many of your questions about how to pay for nursing home care. You can find SHIP's number in the blue pages of your phone book or call your local area agency on aging. You can call Medicare directly at 1-800-633-4227.

Some people think that you have to spend yourself down to poverty to qualify which means the spouse will lose his or her home and spend the rest of his or her life in poverty. But federal laws protect enough of your parent's assets so that the one living at home isn't forced into poverty.

There are lawyers who will show you how to qualify for Medicaid even if you have a high income. There are a number of steps you can take to protect your assets several years in advance of your parent needing nursing home care. Even though this may be legally correct, the ethics are very questionable. States will look back over a period of three to five years to see if you have transferred assets to intentionally misuse Medicaid. These state and federal funds are reserved for those who truly need the financial help. Gaming the system hurts us all in the long run. Rule of thumb: If somebody can afford to hire a lawyer to rework his or her finances to exploit Medicaid, that person can afford to take care of his or her parents without putting them on welfare.

Out of Your Pocket

Nearly half of all nursing home residents pay for their care out their own pockets. In 1996, private payments for nursing home care reached just over $30 billion. Half of all residents are discharged within three months while one in five are there for more than a year but less than three years. If an individual stays for a long period of time and spends all of his or her savings, that person usually becomes eligible for Medicaid.

Medi-Gap or Medicare Supplemental Insurance

Chances are your parents have been paying for a supplemental insurance policy to their Medicare. These policies are commonly referred to as Medi-gap policies because they fill in the gaps between what Medicare pays and whatever is the actual bill from a doctor or hospital. Most plans will also help with the gap between what the nursing home charges and Medicare pays. These Medi-gap policies do *not* pay the full bill.

Veterans Nursing Homes

My dad, a World War II veteran, calls me at least twice a year when he's paying his Medi-gap insurance policy and asks me, "Are you sure I need this? Can't I just go into the Veterans Home and then I won't have to pay anything?" And I always say, "No, Dad. There are millions of veterans out there just like you. There simply aren't enough beds. You have to qualify to get in and they're looking for people with pretty low incomes." Even though the Department of Veterans Affairs provides long-term care services for thousands of veterans, it isn't free. See Chapter 22, "The *Saving Private Ryan* Generation," for more information on services for veterans.

Medicare Managed Care

If your parent has opted out of the traditional, fee-for-service Medicare and into a Medicare managed-care plan, you should know that the managed-care organization must offer your parent the same benefits as those offered under traditional Medicare. This is the minimum the managed-care plan must provide. Check with your parent's plan to see if it covers anything more than the minimum.

Medicaid Waiver Programs

Most states have received waivers from the federal government to offer people who qualify for Medicaid *and* are certified as eligible for nursing home care a choice to either go into a nursing home or remain at home. If someone chooses to stay at home, the state will pay a large portion of the home health care and medical services your parent will need. Every state has its own set of rules. Call your local area agency on aging to find out how to qualify.

So there you have it. If you've learned anything, I hope it's that you are no longer among the misguided who think that Medicare covers your parent's nursing home stay.

Sage Source

There are 131 Veterans Administration-run nursing homes in the country. To find out about one near you and if you are eligible, call 1-800-827-1000 or go to www.va.gov.

Your entire family—parents and siblings—should have a serious discussion on how to financially prepare for nursing home care. If your mom is 85 years old, she has a 50-50 chance of needing nursing home care. With those kinds of odds and the level of expense we're talking about, you can't afford to go merrily along hoping for the best. Some families are pitching in to buy long-term care insurance for their parents while they're in their 60s when it's more affordable. It's not such a high bill to pay when three or four family members are sharing in the cost. For more on long-term care insurance, see Chapter 23, "Beating Out-of-Pocket Expenses."

Targeting Your Search

If you live in a rural area or small town, searching for a nursing home might not be that difficult because you don't have that many choices. But if you do have a good number to choose from, here are five criteria that can help you narrow your search:

1. **Location.** If possible, find a home that is close to family, friends, and your mom or dad's medical specialists so that visits will be convenient.

2. **Availability.** Some homes have waiting lists so depending upon your time constraints, this is the first question you'll need to ask when you call around. No sense spending an hour interviewing an admissions director to find out that the facility can't take your Mom for another six months and she needs it in a week.

3. **Special care needs.** If your parent has Alzheimer's disease, end-stage renal disease requiring dialysis, or requires a ventilator, he or she needs specialized services and staff. Not all homes offer this type of care, so limit your search to those that have it, if this is what your parent needs.

4. **Medicare or Medicaid certified.** If your mom is approved by Medicare for a short stay, you'll need to ask if the home is Medicare certified. If it is not, it can't take your Mom unless you've won the lottery and want to pick up the tab yourself. If Mom is a Medicaid beneficiary, you'll need to ask if the home has been approved by the state to accept Medicaid patients. Nursing homes set aside a certain number of beds for Medicare and Medicaid residents and the beds fill up quickly. If Mom starts off as a private-pay resident but during the course of a long stay becomes a Medicaid beneficiary, be forewarned that the nursing home does *not* have to offer her a bed. Find out early what its policy is regarding this circumstance. You don't want Mom having to transfer if she is happy with the care and has come to like where she's living.

5. **Cultural and religious preferences.** Some nursing homes are run by religious organizations and are often referred to as "faith-based." Though many of these non-profit homes were founded by a particular religious group many welcome people from other faiths. If religion, culture, or a bilingual staff is important to your mom or dad, then you might want to target these types of homes for your search.

Silver Lining

Although all of us hope that our parents won't need to go to a nursing home, it is far better to talk about the circumstances that might lead to this decision while your parents are healthy. It's also wise to check out two or three nursing homes *before* there's a crisis. Finding a home days before a hospital is about to discharge your parent is the worst time to make an informed, compassionate decision.

Doing the Research

If you've recently gone through the ordeal of finding a college or training school for your kids, you know what it's like to sort through loads of material on schools, applications, scholarships, and loan applications. Well, here you go again. Get yourself an expandable folder and set up the following subjects:

1. Parent's medical records
2. Parent's social security number and Medicare data

3. Medi-gap policy papers

4. A folder on each nursing home you're interested in, including the name, phone number, person you talked to, the home's promotional materials, and the results of your site visit and/or interview

5. Your notes from the Nursing Home Site Visit Guide (see Appendix C, "Dr. Rhodes Nursing Home Navigator"), and any other reports on the facilities you're considering

6. Contact list of all agency resources in your community (long-term care ombudsman, area agency on aging, and so on)

Consolidating this information and having it on hand when you're making calls will help you remain organized and stay focused. It's very easy to become overwhelmed, especially if you're conducting this search under the emotional stress of a medical crisis with your parent.

On Becoming a Detective

There are plenty of clues and information on nursing homes that can tell you whether or not they're worthy of taking care of your mom and dad. Just looking over glossy brochures and taking a guided tour isn't going to cut it. Some people spend more time and research buying their car then picking a nursing home! But not you. Here are my best undercover detective tips.

Sage Source

Get the latest survey inspection report on any nursing home in the country by going to www.medicare.gov. Click on Nursing Home Compare and you can search for homes by name or location. Some states are providing even more detailed information on nursing homes on the Web, so also check out your state's official Web site.)

Your first stop is the Internet. The federal government at www.medicare.gov offers you the results of the latest inspection report of every nursing home in the country. Every year nurses from your state visit the home to determine how well the facility meets federal and state requirements for health and safety. Based upon these findings, the report will show you how and what kind of deficiencies the home had at the time of the inspection. All you have to do is enter the name of the home and bang—you get the major results of the inspection. Or you can search for homes by county so you can compare the home you're looking at with others.

Your second stop is to the local ombudsman office. If you used the Medicare Web site you will be given the name and phone number of the local ombudsman (see Chapter 12, "Living in the Community: Services and Transportation," for more on the role of the ombudsman). You can also call your local area agency on aging to get the number.

Here's a list of questions you should ask the local ombudsman:

- Has there ever been a ban on admissions at the home? (If so, why and when?)
- Is there an active family and residents council at the home?
- What kind of inspection reports do they routinely get from state and federal surveyors? (Probe for whether or not they're above or below average.)
- What can you tell me about this nursing home in general? (Ombudsmen are not allowed to recommend one nursing home over another, so don't try pushing him or her for an opinion.)

If you obtained a report on the nursing home from the Medicare Web site, ask the ombudsman to explain it to you.

Your third stop is with hospital social workers. Chances are your mom or dad will be entering a nursing home directly from the hospital or soon after, so you'll have a chance to talk with the social workers. Ask if they have many admissions from the nursing home that you're considering and their impression of the kind of care these patients get. Ask if they are aware of any outstanding problems or complaints about the home.

The final stop is at the nursing home itself. Visit the home at least twice, once during the day and once in the evening. It's really not to your advantage to make a surprise visit—leave that to the inspectors. You'll find my Nursing Home Navigator in Appendix C. Tear it out and make copies for every home you visit. The Guide suggests questions you should ask, things to look for, and tips on how to read between the lines.

Watch What You Agree To

Just like the old college days, you will need to complete an application for the nursing home, and you'll be required to send other documents: A physician will have to certify that your parent really needs nursing home care, you'll need documentation as to how Mom or Dad's care will be paid, as well as any legal documents such as advance directives, a living will, a durable power of attorney for health care, and/or a power of attorney.

Mom or Dad's physician will need to fill out a pre-admission screening form regarding any history of mental illness or mental retardation to assure that the home provides you parent specialized care if needed for either of these conditions. Make sure you take steps to have the admission pre-authorized by any insurance carrier involved in your mom or dad's care. If this admission isn't okay with the insurance carrier before your parent enters the home, you'll get socked with a pretty hefty bill. The nursing home can advise you on those steps.

Senior Alert

Don't waive your rights to Medicare or Medicaid benefits. Nursing homes prefer residents who are private pay—the homes get paid more and have no hassles. But it's illegal for a nursing home to ask you in writing or verbally to *not* apply for Medicare or Medicaid reimbursement for your parent's care. If a home asks you to do that, talk to the local ombudsman and start looking for another home.

Senior Alert

Your parent—not you—should sign the nursing home agreement. There will be language that identifies the person who signs the document as being responsible for all bills. Unless your parent is legally declared incompetent (unable to make decisions) don't sign it and become liable for payments that your parent can't make.

Don't sign on the dotted line until you've really taken the time to carefully read the admissions agreement. Nursing homes must provide you with a fee schedule of what is covered under their basic rate and extra charges for personal services like haircuts, manicures, telephone, or dry cleaning. The basic rate is usually referred to as the per diem charge, meaning the charge per day. Make sure the home spells out what is being covered by Medicare, Medicaid, Medi-gap, Medicare managed care or long-term care insurance and for *how long*. Also ask the home what its policy is when a resident has spent all of his or her private dollars and subsequently becomes a Medicaid beneficiary. Does the resident have to leave?

The law also protects you and your siblings from being financially liable for your parent's care. It's illegal for the nursing home to require this of you as a condition of admission to the facility. Also avoid any advance payments to the home. Medicare rules prohibit nursing homes from requiring you to pay an advance unless it is absolutely, positively clear that Medicare will *not* pay for the care.

Here are some questions you should ask before signing the admissions agreement:

- How much do you charge per day? What's included?
- How do my parent's records remain confidential?
- Are pharmacy services made available? Who prescribes? Who pays?
- What are the facility and state rules for transferring my parent from the home to the hospital or other medical facility?
- If my mom or dad is in the hospital, how long do you hold the bed at the nursing home and how does my parent's per diem rate change?

- What are your billing practices? Are there late charges? If my mom or dad should go on Medicaid, will anything change regarding his or her care or residency at the facility?

- What are your rules and policies regarding personal fund accounts (small amounts of money your parent has access to for incidental spending)?

At the time of admission, you will receive a packet of information on how to apply for Medicaid and Medicare, a resident's bill of rights, a description of your parent's legal rights, how to file a complaint, how to accept or refuse medical or surgical treatment, and how to contact the physician providing care to your parent at the nursing home. Be sure to take the time to read these materials.

The Least You Need to Know

- Approximately 4 percent of those 65 years and older are in nursing homes in the United States. The average resident is at least 85 years old and has a chronic, debilitating condition.

- Don't count on Medicare to pay for your parent's nursing home care: In general, Medicare pays for less than 10 percent of all nursing home bills, and certain restrictions apply.

- Medicaid is the state-run program that pays for nursing home care if your parent has a low income and qualifies.

- There are other options in paying for nursing home care, including Medigap or Medicare supplemental insurance, Medicare managed care, and Medicaid waiver programs.

- When researching nursing homes, it's important to do your homework. Your local ombudsman can answer any questions you may have. The Medicare Web site (www.medicare.gov) is another excellent resource.

- Before signing any admissions agreement, make sure you study it carefully and know exactly what you're agreeing to.

Chapter 16

Living in a Nursing Home

In This Chapter

- Easing the transition
- Who's on staff at the nursing home?
- The kind of care you can expect
- Making your visits count: identifying and solving problems
- Your parent's rights at the nursing home
- Showing your appreciation

Now that your parent is living in a nursing home, you'll need to know what to expect and how to make Mom or Dad's new living arrangement the best for both of you. Nursing homes are a world unto themselves. At first, both you and your parent might feel like foreigners. You won't know the routine or who is responsible for what. The schedule might seem overwhelming, and even though the home will try hard to make you feel "at home," your parent is now a part of group living.

My goal in this chapter is to get you past the tourist feeling and help you both feel comfortable about the nursing home.

First Things First: Assessing Your Parent's Care

By law, nursing homes are required to make a thorough assessment of your mom within two weeks of admission. This exam should cover her level of mobility, skin condition, medical and mental status, nutritional and rehabilitation needs, drug therapy, dental condition, daily habits, and potential to participate in various activities offered at the home. Based upon this assessment, a team—including the doctor, nurse, nursing assistants, social worker, and any specialized therapists your mom might need—meet to develop a care plan.

A good home will include both you and your mom in the care plan. Let the social worker and administrator know that you would want to be consulted in the team's development of the care plan. Offer to be part of the team meeting or interviewed by a member of the care planning team. Ask to see the final care plan. Look it over to make sure that Mom's special needs are being met—such as if she has kidney disease, Alzheimer's disease, or is dependent on a ventilator. The nursing home's physician will order the care plan into effect. In turn, the charge nurse and nursing assistants should follow this care plan and record their progress accordingly. These plans are also updated throughout the year. Request the home to send you updated copies of the plan.

Senior Alert

According to state and federal reports, the most frequent violation of nursing homes is *not* completing a care plan for each resident. Insist that this be done within the first two weeks of your parent's admission. It's your one guarantee that a concrete, written plan of action has been developed for everyone to follow. Get a copy, so that you, too, can keep track of your parent's progress.

Easing the Adjustment Period

Just like anyone who embarks on a new venture in life, your mom will go through an adjustment period as a result of living in an institutional setting. No matter how hard they try to make the nursing home look like a home, it's still an institutional life with lots of strangers and routines that are not familiar to your mom. So don't be surprised that, on your first few visits, she seems disoriented and confused. You, too, will go through a roller coaster of emotions, from feeling guilty to feeling relieved that she's getting around-the-clock care.

Here are some things you can do to ease the transition:

- Make sure you visit the nursing home with Mom *before* the day of admission.
- Bring personal belongings and small furniture items that Mom is attached to— let them be her choice.

- Bring a photo of Mom with a brief description of what she's done, her hobbies and family member names to have placed on her door for staff to see.

- Bring family photos, wall hangings that she likes, a calendar, and clock.

- Put in writing and share with staff a list of your mom's routines: when she eats breakfast, lunch, and dinner, special dietary needs, bathing habits, whether she's a morning or night person, her favorite TV shows, time of day she goes to bed, and religious practices.

- Meet with the social worker and ask him or her to look in on your mom the first few weeks and let you know how she is emotionally adjusting to the move.

- Since most nursing homes offer semiprivate rooms, encourage the home to match up your mom with a roommate with whom she'll likely be compatible.

- Get to know your mom's roommate. If after a six-week trial period, your mom and the roommate are a worse match than Tony Randall and Jack Klugman in *The Odd Couple,* go to the administrator and see what can be done to find your mom a new roommate.

A Rundown of the Major Players

As you can well imagine, nursing homes have a lot going on. They're caring for very sick and frail people who, in most instances, aren't able to do for themselves. Over half the residents are incontinent and/or suffer from dementia. So the demands are high for one-on-one attention. Who can your mom count on?

There will be at least one medical director who is a physician and will be on 24-hour call. The doctor is required by law to see your mom at least once every 60 days. With that much leeway, you won't see doctors roaming the halls like they do in hospitals or the television show *ER.* Instead, you'll find nurses (why else would they call them *nursing* homes) overseeing and providing the care. The registered nurses are responsible for giving out medications, supervising nursing assistants, and doing paperwork.

Most of the care given to your mom is provided by certified nursing assistants (CNAs). They're the ones helping her get dressed, bathed, groomed, and showered. They'll help her get to the toilet, bring meals, and reposition her in bed. They are also the ones to alert the nurses to potential problems. Nursing assistants must be certified, which means they've taken courses and passed a state exam to prove that they are competent. Most homes also require a police background check. Nursing homes must also check whether or not an aide is listed on a state registry that keeps track of nurse aides who have been found guilty of abuse or neglect.

Nursing homes also have a social worker who can help you with financial and legal matters, or a transfer to another home or the hospital. They can also help your mom with her emotional needs (either arising from the move or ongoing mental health needs), and work with the nursing staff to identify ways to meet any of your mom's unique needs.

Silver Lining

If you have a complaint or some issue that you've tried to work out at the nursing home and it wasn't resolved, the ombudsman can help. It's the ombudsman's job to help resolve conflicts and, if you prefer, he or she will keep things confidential. The ombudsman can also help you better understand your parent's rights in the nursing home. The name and number of the ombudsman is posted on a bulletin board at the nursing home as required by law. They are available to you on an as-needed basis.

Nursing homes, of course, have a licensed administrator and most homes either employ or have contracts with different kinds of therapists (such as physical, occupational, speech, and music therapists). The home should also have a full-time recreation director.

Sage Source

The National Citizen's Coalition for Nursing Home Reform has excellent information on resident's rights and the laws that oversee nursing homes (www.nccnhr.org or 202-332-2275). The Administration on Aging has an excellent Web site that provides you with a list of area agencies on aging and ombudsmen. It also has a resource section with over 200 links (www. aoa.gov, or call their Elder Locator at 1-800-677-1116).

All homes also have family resident councils, consisting of family members and residents, that usually meet every month. Councils sponsor activities at the home and discuss ways to continuously improve to the quality of life at the home. Get to know the members on the council and if you can, attend a meeting. They can give you a real sense of what's going on at the nursing home and whom you should get to know.

The Kind of Care You Should Expect

Nursing homes must meet minimum standards of care required by state and federal laws. A team of nurses, usually referred to as surveyors, are sent in to survey and inspect the home every 12 to 15 months to make sure that they are meeting those standards. Here's what you should know about the care your parent will receive:

- **Independence.** Nursing homes are supposed to help your Dad remain as independent as possible in performing daily tasks such as bathing, walking, eating, using the toilet, and speaking. Unless he has a medical condition that will cause him to deteriorate no matter what, the home's job is to keep him from diminishing for as long as possible.

- **Incontinence.** If your mom is incontinent (urinates involuntarily), the first response of the home should not be to just put her on a catheter (a tube inserted into the bladder that dispenses urine into a bag). The home should try a bladder training program first; if that isn't effective, it must keep your mom dry and prevent urinary tract infections.

- **Bed or pressure sores.** Here's something you have to be vigilant about. Because your mom's skin is more fragile, and she isn't moving around as much, she is susceptible to getting bruises from the pressure of her body's weight against her bed or a chair. This is especially true around bony areas like her tailbone, elbows, and heels. Reddened areas around the skin are the first sign. If these are not attended to Mom can end up with an open sore that can even expose the bone. At that stage, they are very stubborn to treat and are vulnerable to deadly infection.

  Sometimes, bed sores are due to lack of turning someone who is bedridden, letting someone lay in urine for too long, or not taking care of the person's skin. As secretary of aging, I investigated several cases of outright neglect of nursing home patients who had such horrible bed sores that they died.

Geri-Fact

Most homes try very hard to prevent bed sores, but it's something you should always be on guard for. Let the nurse know as soon as you see any redness on your parent's skin. You can help by giving your mom a massage on your visit and asking the nurse how you can be helpful with Mom's skin care.

- **Restraints.** Nursing homes can't strap your mom to her bed or a chair, place her in a chair that she can't get out of, or use bed rails that she can't undo herself. Nor can they chemically restrain her by giving her drugs that sedate her all day long so she's not bothering anyone. Restraints cannot be used for disciplinary reasons or staff convenience. On the other hand, you may worry that if your mom falls out of bed she may break her hip. Ask the nursing home to share with you their practices on restraints and what alternatives they use to keep the patients from harming themselves.

- **Medications.** Nursing homes must provide pharmacy services to each resident, but that doesn't mean the home pays for the prescriptions. Remember,

Medicare currently doesn't cover prescriptions, so unless your mom has special insurance, prescriptions are paid out of pocket. The nursing home also employs a pharmacist who reviews your mom's drug regimen at least once a month and alerts the doctor and nurse of any problems. A home is allowed no more than a 5 percent error rate in dispensing medications. Psychotropic drugs (mind-altering) should be prescribed only if clinically proven by a physician to be necessary. See Chapter 8, "Pills and Your Parents."

- **Therapies.** The facility is required to offer your mom range-of-motion exercises to keep her joints and limbs limber, usually performed by a physical therapist. Mom should also receive dental, vision, and hearing treatment along with any assistive devices to help maintain her functioning. Mental health therapy, including help with psychosocial problems as a result of difficulties in adjusting to nursing home life, should also be offered. If your mom appears depressed, let the nurse know so that a consult can be arranged.

- **Nutrition and hydration.** Believe it or not, your mom is vulnerable to malnutrition and dehydration even in the nursing home. In fact a recent study by The Commonwealth Fund, found that one third of the 1.6 million nursing home residents in the United States may suffer from malnutrition and dehydration! The study contends that this is due in large part to lack of staff. So, if your mom can't feed herself, has lost her appetite (people begin losing their sense of taste and smell in their 60s), is depressed, or if the home isn't closely monitoring how much she's eating when they drop off her dinner tray, she can suffer from malnutrition. This can lead to confusion and a reduced immune system. Watch for unexplained weight loss. Let the nurses know that you want the aides to encourage your mom to eat and perhaps give her supplements. On your visits, be sure to check on whether or not she has access to fresh water. When you call her, be sure to ask her when she had her last drink of water and what she ate during her most recent meal.

Senior Alert

If your mom has extreme difficulty in feeding herself, the home might recommend tube feeding. This option should be used only as an absolute last resort. Make sure it's not being recommended purely as a means of staff convenience and not in the best interest of your mother.

If your mom is taking medications, the staff needs to make sure she's getting enough fresh water throughout the day because some medications can dehydrate her. She also might be restricting her own fluids because she finds it too difficult to get to the bathroom or she doesn't want to void in her adult brief. Being dehydrated can be very dangerous. So be on the lookout.

Make Your Visits Count

Besides the emotional support you'll give your dad by coming to see him, you can become his best advocate. How? By staying on top of his care. You don't need to be a doctor or nurse to pick up telltale signs that something's amiss. Following is my list of what should catch your attention every time you visit. Share this with other family members and if none of you lives near your dad's nursing home then find a local volunteer—either through a senior center, church, or synagogue who'll make frequent visits for you. Residents who are visited regularly by family and friends are at a definite advantage. Don't let your dad be on the losing side.

Making Your Nursing Home Visit Count: What to Look For

- Any redness or bruises on the skin especially near bony areas like the tailbone, heels, and elbows? You're checking for bed or pressure sores.

- Any weight loss, change in appetite, sores in the mouth, problems with dentures, chewing, or extremely thirsty? You're checking for malnutrition and dehydration.

- Any ingrown toenails, infections, bunions, uncut nails on the feet? You're checking for potential serious infections and problems in walking, especially if your parent is diabetic. These could also be signs of poor care.

- Poorly kept hair, beard, clothing not clean or pressed, body odor, wet adult briefs, unclean sheets? These are signs of poor care and can lead to pressure sores, infections, and depression.

- Takes too long for calls to be answered, aides frequently tell you, "Sorry, we're short-staffed today," meal trays are served late, no fresh water in the room, aides assigned to more residents than they can reasonably handle? These are signs of poor care due to lack of staff.

- Clothes or belongings missing? Periodically check closets and drawers to make sure that your parent isn't missing any personal items.

- Seems like every time you turn around there's a new director of nursing or head nurse, or your dad rarely has the same nursing aide from one week to the next? Staff morale seems pretty low? It won't take long for high staff turnover rates to spill over into poor care.

What to Do on Your Visits

Besides staying on top of your parent's care, there are a number of things you can do to make your visit with your mom or dad a productive and pleasant one. Here are some suggestions:

- Listen to your parent's complaints. If they are frequent and consistent, check into it. If Dad complains about food, visit during meal times; if it's about his roommate, get to know the roommate and determine if things can be worked out or not; if the complaint is about a certain staff person, visit when that person is on shift. Assess these complaints and work with the nurse supervisor to correct the problem.

- Take your parent out for brief excursions, if possible. If Mom can leave her room, take her to a quiet visiting area; if the weather's nice, head for an outside garden area.

- If you bring the kids or a family pet, arrange an activity that your dad can do with the kids or Lassie. My son at the age of eight used to play checkers with a resident of a nursing home. Dr. Jenkins had forgotten much of the game and Matt knew little of it but they had a great time.

- Bring a small gift when you come so Dad can remember you came (candy is not a good idea), mark the calendar to show him you were there, hug him, hold hands, and when you enter the room, announce who you are, "Hi Dad, it's your daughter Linda." (I always add, "You know, your *favorite* daughter," just to rattle my sister.) You could also bring a Polaroid camera and take pictures of your visit to leave behind.

- Always end your visit by checking in with a staff member. Let him or her know you were there, that you appreciate his or her help; share some tidbit about Dad and ask the staff member for of any insights he or she has about your dad's health. Don't stick to one staff member: take turns with the administrator, head nurse, social worker, recreation director, physical therapist, and various nurse aides. You'll learn more about your dad, and more people will know how much you care.

- If you live out of town, visit through frequent phone calls. If you can live by a schedule, then make a certain day a visiting day by calling on a set day, like Sunday afternoons. Sending a video of family events or just for the fun of it, is also a good way to reinforce that your parent is still part of the family. You'll need to make sure that someone at the home, perhaps the activities director, will play the video for your parent. And of course, there's always the mail. Older people love to receive letters and postcards letting them know you're thinking of them. If your parent is hard of hearing, getting a letter in the mail may be easier for both of you than talking on the phone.

Silver Lining

Many nursing homes throughout the country are discovering ways to make the home feel like less of an institution. Some offer pet therapy in partnership with the local humane society, in which gentle dogs and cats are brought in for the residents to hold and pet. Some facilities even have their own resident dog or cat! Birds are heard chirping in cages amidst plants throughout many facilities. Homes are also changing the work environment to increase staff morale, and improving the decor of the facility to make everyone feel at home and part of a family. If your parent's facility doesn't offer such programs, meet with the family resident council and initiate them!

Your Parent's Rights

Nursing homes must meet stringent standards of care by law if they are to participate in Medicare or Medicaid. However, don't assume that just because the laws are on the books that there are enough people overseeing the laws. In Appendix D, "Nursing Home Bill of Rights," you'll find a list that outlines your parent's rights when living at a nursing home.

If you have complaints or suspect abuse, neglect, or exploitation of your parent, you can go to the ombudsman or you can call the elder abuse hotline run by your local area agency on aging listed in the phone book. People there have the expertise to confidentially look into your complaint and determine what must be done.

If you visit your parent and discover that Mom or Dad has fallen or had any other accident and you were *not* notified, ask to see the accident report. According to law, the home must notify you if your parent has suffered *any* accident. Find out the circumstances. Sometimes accidents do happen and it was unavoidable. But if something doesn't feel right about the home's story, your parent refutes it or is unusually quiet about it, or these sort of accidents seem all too frequent at the home (ask to see the home's *monthly* accident report), see the ombudsman and report the incident. Visit your dad at different times of the day, so that you get a better sense of who cares for him during various shifts. If at all possible, attend a few resident council meetings; you'll find out what's working and what's not.

Appreciate the Staff

Even though I've warned you about the things you should watch for in a nursing home, the vast majority of homes are very good. Given your parent's condition, being cared for at a facility is probably much better for Mom or Dad than being cared for at home. As difficult as the decision was for me to place Grandma into a nursing home, I know it was the best for her. The care she required was simply beyond us.

Geri-Fact

According to the U.S. Department of Labor, nursing assistants in nursing homes have one of the highest injury rates of any workers in the United States. They sustain these injuries from caring for residents (lifting) and from assaults by residents! This doesn't include the verbal abuse many nursing assistants endure on a daily basis.

Caring for older, frail people is both rewarding and very difficult. I've personally interviewed over 700 nurse's aides asking them what was important to them in the workplace. The word *respect* came out loud and clear. They want to be respected by both management and families for their knowledge, their hard work, and for going the extra mile to make your parent feel loved. Most see caring for the el-derly as a calling, especially among the older workers. They feel rewarded when they've made someone smile, given first-rate care, and made your dad feel like family. You should know that the salary for nursing assistants is extremely low. Your teenager can make as much behind a retail counter at the mall. So, whenever you can show staff respect and thank them, do it.

The Least You Need to Know

- Within the first two weeks of your parent's admission, the home must do a complete workup on your parent and develop a plan of care. Get a copy.

- There is an ombudsman for every nursing home who can help you re-solve any conflicts or problems on your parent's behalf. The ombuds-man's name and phone number must be openly posted at the facility.

- Do more than just pass the time on a visit. Learn how to assess your parent's care, pick up warning signs, and help with some of the care yourself.

- Most of the care given to residents is given by nursing assistants—not registered nurses or doctors.

- Caring for older, frail people is both rewarding and difficult. Remember to show your appreciation to the staff.

Part 4

Caregiving: Coming to Live with You

Caregiving in the home—whether it's raising kids, caring for an ailing spouse, or caring for your parents—is never easy. Yet it can be one of the most rewarding things you'll ever do. You must be very honest with yourself, however, on what it takes to care for someone. This part of the book helps you size up your life—work, family, ability, and resources—so that you can make a balanced and realistic decision to bring your parent in to live with you.

Once you've made the decision and it's a go, you'll be given a crash course on the ins and outs of caregiving. We also show you how to take care of yourself. Stretching yourself too thin is an all too common health hazard among caregivers. Whether your parents live with you or not, be sure to read Chapter 20, "End-of-Life Matters and Hospice." Coming to terms with dying is a milestone we must all reach with our parents and ourselves. You'll learn how hospice care can get you there.

Chapter 17

Are You Up for This?

In This Chapter

- Assessing your parent's needs—and yours
- How will being a caregiver affect your work and family life?
- Sizing up the costs and other factors
- Getting the entire family involved by calling a family meeting
- Making the decision to be a caregiver

There's good reason for the saying, "Love is blind." Just ask any parent of a teenager. And I'm sure you've looked back on a relationship or two yourself and thought, "What was I thinking?"

Now that we're on this love theme, I'm going to guess that you really love your parents. Chances are you wouldn't have bothered buying this book if you didn't care about their welfare. For most of us the child-parent bond yields a love that is unconditional. So when your mom and dad reach a point in their lives where they need you to take care of them, your first instinct is an unconditional yes. But blindly jumping into a caregiving role with your parents to prove your love can result in a pretty rough landing. The goal of this chapter is to take the blinders off and give you as soft a landing as possible.

What Does Your Parent Need?

Hopefully, your parent has had a geriatric assessment (see Chapter 7, "Managing the Health Care Maze—Even from a Distance") so that you are fully aware of their needs. But even if you are, translating medical needs into everyday life is another story. So before you totally commit to caring for Mom or Dad at home, do your own assessment.

Begin your assessment by asking yourself how much help your dad needs with the activities of daily living. Use the following chart to estimate how much time is needed and who will be the caregiver for each of the following functions:

Activity	Amount of Time?	Caregiver?
Eating (Will you have to prepare all meals? Is he able to feed himself? Is he on a special diet?)		
Bathing (Will he need assistance showering? Shaving? Help with daily grooming?)		
Using the toilet (Will he need help going to and from the bathroom? Is he incontinent?)		
Dressing (Can he get dressed on his own?)		
Medications (Will he need to be reminded or will you need to administer them?)		
Transporting (How often will he need to go to the doctors? Therapists? Will you do the scheduling?)		
In-home therapies (Any daily therapies? What daily medical care does he need?)		
Finances (Will you be taking over all of his finances? Bill paying?)		
Supervision (Can he safely be left alone or is he confused, prone to wander or fall? Does he not sleep at night?)		

Don't underestimate how much work each of these activities require. If your dad is in the early stages of a disease, especially Alzheimer's, think through what you'll be doing to care for him down the line. Caring for your parent can be extremely rewarding. Taking care of Grandma (my children's great grandmother) for a year was an experience filled with "Kodak moments" and deeply cherished memories for me. I wouldn't trade that year for anything. But caring for her was not without hardships. At the end of the year, she suffered two strokes and acute dementia. I had to learn to let go and place her in a setting that could meet her demanding physical needs better than I could. You'll need to strike a balance between what's good for your parent and what you are able to do. It also means knowing what is good for you and your own family.

Sizing Up Your Life

Now that you have a handle on all of your dad's needs, you need to size up a few things before you take the caregiving plunge.

If you are like most caregivers, you're a woman who has a job outside of the home and a husband, and you're between 40 to 60 years old. And some of you are pulling triple duty: One out of four caregivers has children at home. Congrats! You get to play a lot of roles in life: Mom, wife, daughter, and employee. Adding the caregiving role of a dependent parent to the mix will affect the balance you might have achieved with your family and work. So before the scales go completely out of whack, let's figure out how to tip the scales in your favor.

Your Work Life

Before you bring Dad home to live with you, take the time to talk to your employer. It's not that you're seeking permission—your employer can actually help you. Many large companies have programs that can assist you in finding services to help you take care of your parent and keep your job humming along. Several companies contract with employers to provide services (most often called "Employee Assistance Programs" (EAP) or "Work/Life" programs). Sometimes the employee directly talks with the contractor and its consultants; in other instances, the employee deals with the employer's Human Resources (HR) office or EAP. Ask your HR or EAP staff if this contracted assistance is available.

If your workplace doesn't cover the service, visit the Web sites of the following companies to get an idea of the kinds of help they offer workers. Be sure to share this information with your company:

- **Child and Elder Care Insights, Inc.,** offers two trademarked databases to assist employees—CHILDBASE and ELDERBASE. Employees can access the databases by calling the company or by going online. Consultants can provide individualized assistance in a variety of ways: by phone, by responding to an e-mail request, and by virtual communication online. Contact them at 216-356-2900 or www.carereports.com.

- **Dependent Care Connection, Inc.,** offers counseling, referral, and educational service to employees, both by phone and online. Dependent Care Connection claims 24-hour access to information, uses an employee personal profile to deliver individualized information to the employee, and organizes Web information by specific life events to help employees find information quickly. Contact them at 1-800-873-4636 or www.dcclifecare.com.

- **Ceridian** offers the trademarked **LifeWorks Employee Resource Program** to help employees find solutions to work and personal issues. Employees and their dependents can get help with personal problems, child and elder care resources, managing stress and change, legal and financial issues, and locating help in their own communities. Contact them at 1-800-788-1949 (Ceridian) or 1-800-635-0606 (LifeWorks), or www.ceridianperformance.com.

Silver Lining

Your employer may offer other benefits, such as helping you pay for adult day care. You may be able to work out a flexible schedule, such as working four 10-hour days. Maybe you could stretch vacation time into long weekends, or share your job with a new Mom who also wants to work flexible hours. Many employers also allow their employees to work at home ("telecommute") at least part of the work week.

Be up front with your boss, letting him or her know how you plan to manage your work. Go on the offensive and present a plan that shows how you can meet your job objectives and meet your new caregiving demands. Don't let missed meetings, coming in late, or making long-distance calls on company time be the reason you finally let the boss know why you've fallen behind.

No matter how noble it is that you're taking care of your parent, you do have a responsibility to your co-workers in getting your job done. And you have the right to both enjoy and further your career. The only way you can achieve all of this is to honestly assess what you can humanly do to care for your dad and still maintain your job and other commitments. To do this you'll need to enlist help (paid and family members), identify tasks and activities that someone else can do or that you can take a break from, and set some boundaries where family members respect your time at work. In other words, ditch your Wonder Woman cape. You can't do it all. Nor should you!

Silver Lining

In 1993, Congress passed the Family and Medical Leave Act (FMLA). Employers with 50 or more employees must allow their workers at least 12 weeks of *unpaid* leave for a family member who is seriously ill. The law defines family member as the worker's spouse, parent, or child. If you are caring for your in-law or grandparent, the law doesn't apply. To qualify, you must have worked for the company an average of 24 hours or more per week for at least one year. Your company must give you full health benefits during your leave, and you're entitled to get your old job back or another position with equivalent duties, same salary and benefits.

For more details on FMLA, visit the U.S. Department of Labor Web site at www.dol.gov. Click onto "Laws and Regulations" and enter FMLA at the search button.

Your Family Life

Unless you live alone, the decision for bringing Mom home to stay shouldn't be a command decision that you make and simply announce to your family. Your spouse and kids, if they live with you, should be part of this decision. The whole family will be greatly affected by your mom or dad coming to live with you. Even if everyone is happy about the idea and supportive, relationships are going to be tested. Kids aren't going to get your undivided attention. You'll feel guilty missing that baseball game. Your husband will need to pitch in more and may find you stressed out and not know how to respond. And there you are: feeling pulled in all directions.

So before you make this life-changing decision, assess your family resources: What are your kids' needs? How much can your husband help given his work demands? What are the strengths of your marriage? What are the weaknesses? What can your siblings do? How is your relationship with your parent? (Is it rocky? Will it disrupt an

Geri-Fact

A national survey by the National Family Caregiver's Association found that the most frequently reported frustration felt by caregivers—76 percent—was the lack of consistent help from other family members.

otherwise harmonious home?) How does your parent get along with your spouse? If you have teenagers or adult children, how can they help? Be realistic as to how your loved ones are going to respond to this new challenge.

If you'll be caring for a parent who has Alzheimer's disease, make sure that everyone understands the nature and course of the disease. Children can become very frightened of Grandma if they don't understand what's going on. And though this is part of life, you'll need to guide your children through the debilitating side of growing old.

Your Ability

This might be the hardest assignment of all. On one hand, you'll be surprised at the inner resources you have when you rise to the occasion. On the other hand, you may find that you are definitely over your head trying to meet your mom's physical, emotional, and mental health needs along with all of your family and work obligations. Take stock of your weaknesses and the things that really rattle you. Determine if any of these factors are going to be frequent hot-button issues for you when you care for your parent.

Geri-Fact

According to the National Family Caregiver Association's study of caregivers, 70 percent said that one of the most positive outcomes of their caregiving experience was finding the inner strength they didn't know they had.

Say, for instance, your mom has several chronic conditions that require a great deal of scheduling, transporting, and organizing treatments. However, you're one of those free spirits who hates day planners and has yet to replace the battery in your watch. You'll need to enlist someone to either create order in your life or take over that element of your mom's care. If you're squeamish—can't handle insulin shots, incontinence, or changing dressings, and that is what your parent needs on a daily basis—you really need to ask yourself, if you can do this.

If you aren't realistic going into this, then you'll be at risk of becoming resentful or feeling trapped. Not a good place to be.

Sizing Up Your Resources

Now that you've sized up your life, you need to carefully assess the resources you have available to take care of your parent. Following are some of the resources you should consider.

Space

The first question you'll need to answer is, where will Mom stay? Which room will be hers? If you don't have a spare room, do you have the resources to do a bit of remodeling? One of the more common redesign strategies to accommodate a parent is to make the dining room into a bedroom. There are two benefits: the dining room is usually on the first floor, the same floor as a bathroom, and it allows the older person to feel part of the coming and going of family life, especially if the person is bedridden. Whatever room you choose, it's best if the bathroom is near your mom or, at the very least, on the same floor. For strategies on making the house safer for an elderly parent, see Chapter 11, "Remaining at Home: Making It Work." There are programs that can assist you with remodeling if you're caring for an aging parent. Call your local area agency on aging to see if you qualify (1-800-677-1116).

Skills and Siblings

Every family has its own unique set of resources that it brings to the table. Think of your family as a skills bank. Some families have nurses, others have insurance agents, lawyers, nursing assistants, plumbers, carpenters, or bankers in the clan. The carpenter can install a ramp, and the plumber can put in a bathroom on the first floor. The insurance agent can keep up with the Medi-gap policy, and so on. Rather then thinking of yourselves as brothers, sisters, and cousins, take a look at the *skills* that you have among you. Besides offering special skills, just about anyone can be a driver. And everybody can take turns watching Mom while you get out of the house for a break. Get everyone to make a list of their skills and what they would like to do to help. Match these up against the needs of your parent and what you need as a caregiver. Then develop a schedule to make use of the resources offered by other family members.

Finances

Taking care of someone at home can be costly. There are a number of community resources that you can tap to assist you, if you qualify. Many of these are identified for you in Chapter 10, "Home Health Care." In Chapter 12, "Living in the Community: Services and Transportation," you're given information on tracking down home health care and homemaker aides. But when it comes to most custodial care, you'll find yourself picking up the tab. Here are some of the costs you'll need to consider when it comes to caring for your parent in your own home:

- Renovation costs (install new bathroom and wheelchair ramps, add safety devices)
- Modifications to the bathroom
- Over-the-counter drugs
- Prescription medications
- Dietary needs, meal preparation
- Disposable supplies (adult briefs for incontinence, egg crate pads for the bed, tissues, moisture-proof pads)

- Transportation services
- Cost of hired help (cleaning service, someone to help with care, someone to stay with the person)
- Cost of adult day care
- Co-pays for any therapies or home health care
- Hearing aids
- Eyeglasses
- Dentures

Hopefully, many of these expenses are covered through your parent's income (Social Security, pensions, and other sources). If, however, your parent's income is modest it may mean that you and other family members will need to pick up the difference. You can also explore community services, Medicaid, and faith-based programs that can help with the costs when your parent has a low or modest income.

Senior Alert

To prevent family conflicts, draft a budget showing what is being spent on your mom's care. A file for bills and receipts can help you keep track of your expenses. Don't assume that everyone in the family knows the costs of caregiving. Your siblings might think that Mom has quite a nest egg, when in fact, she doesn't. Keep the communication channels open.

Holding a Family Meeting

I hope the image that you conjure up when you hear "family meeting" isn't one of Archie Bunker and "Meathead" going at it with Edith trying to keep peace between them. If that describes your family, ask a social worker or some outside, qualified person (parish priest, minister, or rabbi) to facilitate the meeting. Even if everyone has to pitch in to pay for a social worker, it will be well worth the expense.

Why a family meeting? Unless you are an only child and your parent has no living relatives, you owe it to yourself, your parent, and your siblings to have the entire family actively involved in caring for your parent. This can be a very rewarding experience for everyone; it's a time to say thank you to the one who has raised you, to gain closure on the most significant relationship of a lifetime, and to forgive and forget. And quite simply, you'll need the help.

Here's how to have a positive and productive family meeting:

1. Do your homework. Clearly lay out your parent's medical, physical, social, and mental health needs. Share medical reports and doctor's notes on your parent's condition(s) with treatment recommendations.

2. Write up a daily routine that shows a typical day of caregiving so that other family members get a practical sense of what is involved. Use the Activity/Amount of Time/Caregiver chart at the beginning of this chapter.

3. Present a budget identifying your parent's resources and monthly income in one column and the expenses of caregiving in the other column. Identify potential debts.

4. Invite your siblings to the meeting. If in-laws are close and usually participate in other family decisions then it may be appropriate to include them, too. The spouse of the family caregiver should be involved because his or her life is definitely affected by the caregiving situation. Your parent's wishes must be respected. If Mom or Dad is competent, he or she should be involved. You might also want to involve a more distant relative who has expertise in a certain area, like a cousin who is a lawyer or nurse.

5. Create an agenda. Call family members ahead of time and ask them the three most important things they would like to discuss at the meeting. You'll find that many of you will share the same concerns. Determine among you who will facilitate this meeting. That person's job will be to organize the agenda and keep the discussion on task.

6. Chances are most of the family members will have had experiences in being a part of other meetings with basic ground rules. It will probably feel a little strange for your family to act so formal. But it is a safeguard from falling into old patterns of teasing brothers and hair-pulling sisters. Here are some tried-and-true strategies in productive group discussion:

   - No cutting in. Wait until someone is finished talking.

   - When you have something to say, it should reflect what you think, not what you think others think. So start the sentence with "I."

   - No accusations. (As in, "you always side in with him.")

   - Stay focused on your parent's needs. Rally around what's best for Mom.

   - If you're not clear on a point that someone else has said, ask that person to clarify it rather than assume something he or she didn't mean.

   - If you want to make sure you've interpreted what the other person has said, try this approach: "This is what I heard you say .... Is that correct?"

Silver Lining

If all of you live out of town and can't get together for a family meeting (even during a traditional family gathering), try a conference call. It's important that you all share in the decision-making, if at all possible.

At the end of the meeting, the facilitator should wrap up what everyone has decided and check to see if this is what everybody understands as the action plan. Someone should be responsible for writing up the plan of who is going to do what and what was decided at the meeting. Make copies and distribute them among each other.

Making the Decision

If you have been able to go through all of these steps—assessing your parent's needs, his or her resources, your resources, and what other family members are willing to do to help you—you're in a position to make a well-informed decision. Now, you need to have a heart-to-heart talk with the members of your immediate family who will be literally living with this decision. Young children deserve to understand what's going on. With Grandma living with them, the youngsters will soon learn that the whole world doesn't revolve around them. You'll need to be sensitive to their changing needs and their feelings of guilt when they secretly wish that Grandma would just go away or even die. Make your children feel like part of the solution; they, too, can have chores that they enjoy doing to help Grandma.

And then there's your marriage. Don't bludgeon your husband with a guilt stick into accepting this new venture, as if he has nothing to say in the matter. The road of caregiving is filled with compromises which only work if they are made mutually.

The Least You Need to Know

- Caregiving is a family affair. Don't try it as a solo act.

- Do your homework: Assess your parent's needs and match them up with your resources. Anticipate the shortfalls, then plan for them.

- There are ways to balance your work life with your new caregiving responsibilities. The Family and Medical Leave Act can protect you, and many employers offer Employee Assistance Programs and Work/Life programs.

- Call a family meeting to get everyone to rally around taking care of Mom or Dad. If family relations are strained, get a professional facilitator such as a social worker, or ask a priest, rabbi, or minister.

Chapter 18

Caring for Someone at Home: The Basics

In This Chapter

- Before you bring your parent home …
- Creating a bedroom that's not a sick room
- Good nutrition: becoming a chef to seniors
- Making bath time a relaxing and positive experience
- Caregiving tips for handling someone with dementia
- When Mom or Dad is prone to wander

You've made the decision to bring Mom or Dad home to live with you. Or you're playing it smart and figure you'll read this chapter so you'll know what you're in for. Good move. I remember when I decided to bring Grandma home to live with us. Despite all of my training, I was pretty nervous. Here I was pregnant with my first child and before you know it, I'm responsible for another human being. She appeared to have dementia, she was incontinent, and she was clearly malnourished. Lots of questions were running through my mind: How was I going to care for her *and* a new baby? Was I getting myself in over my head? Will we get along with each other?

After a geriatric assessment, it was clear that her dementia was caused by being malnourished and her incontinence was caused by not being able to negotiate steps because of a cataract. So after a month of good food, cataract surgery, and lots of attention, Grandma became a new person. Caring for Lena taught me a great deal and gave me an appreciation of what caregivers endure. There is also a gift of joy that caregivers receive knowing the peace, dignity, and comfort they've made possible for a loved one nearing the end of his or her life. In this chapter I'll share some of the caregiving basics that I learned along the way and some that others recommend, too.

Getting Ready

If you're a parent, remember when you ran around getting the nursery ready, buying a car seat, and taking Lamaze classes? All this to get ready for a tiny eight-pound newcomer to the family household. Even though there's a bit of difference in weight, there should also be a flurry of activity getting the house ready for your elderly newcomer. Here are three major things to consider.

Sage Source

There are some excellent Web sites dedicated to helping caregivers of the elderly. Here are two of the best:

- **CaregiverZone (www.caregiverzone.com).** This excellent site is a one-stop shop for information, services, and resources for caregiving. The site was designed by a social worker in senior services.

- **Caregiver Survival Resources (www.caregiver911.com).** This site is maintained by a couple who have 35 years of professional caregiving experience. The site is easy to use, offers questions and answers on caregiving, links to other resources, and a chat room.

An excellent video series, *Aging Parents: The Family Survival Guide*, tells you all about how to care for your aging parent. It's been endorsed by the National Council on Aging. The cost is $99 (perhaps a local hospital would buy it and loan it out). Check it out on the Web at www.agingparents.com or call 1-888-777-5585.

Organizing the Paperwork

You'll need to gather all of Mom's paperwork: bills, insurance papers, finance papers, and medical records, and then create your own file to keep track of the onslaught of more papers to come your way when you care for her. Chapter 7, "Managing the Health Care Maze—Even from a Distance," provides you with a checklist of what to collect and how to organize it. Be sure to take advantage of the Pill Tracking Chart in Chapter 8, "Pills and Your Parents," if your mom takes multiple medications.

Doctors Orders and Nurse's Notes

If you're bringing your dad home from the hospital, make sure that the doctor and nurse give you complete and understandable instructions on how to care for him. Have them chart out when he is to take his medications, how many pills to take during the day, and whether or not he should take them with food. Dietary needs, exercise regimens, and use of durable medical equipment should be explained to you. Ask for a number that you can call if you think you need added advice or encounter any problems.

Accident-Proofing the House

I really felt schizophrenic when I was caring for both Grandma and my son, Matthew. At one end of the house I was creating obstacles to keep him *out of* trouble, and at the other end I was removing obstacles to keep Grandma from getting *into* trouble. Hopefully, you can be single-minded about this. Chapter 11, "Remaining at Home: Making It Work," gives you all kinds of ideas to create a safe environment for your parent to live alone. Use the same ideas for your home. Here are some additional tips:

- Install amplifiers and lights to alert seniors that the telephone is ringing or someone's ringing the door bell.

- Purchase recliners or seat cushions that make getting in and out of a chair easy.

- Install devices such as motion detectors that alert you that Mom is up at night wandering, especially alerting you if she is opening a door to get outside.

- Remove clutter wherever possible. This is especially helpful if your mom has dementia. Keep things in the bathroom simple, same on the kitchen counter. Hallways and steps should always be clear, especially the pathway to the bathroom.

- Install motion detectors that automatically turn on lights at night, such as in the bathroom and hallways, so Mom doesn't have to fumble around finding a light switch in the dark. Nightlights alone don't provide enough light.

Try to incorporate some of your mom's favorite furniture pieces into your home—even if it doesn't match the decor. If you're a fan of the TV show *Frasier,* just think of his Dad's chair gloriously kept together with duct tape amidst Frasier's pricey furniture.

Your Parent's Bedroom

As your parent's health needs increase, the bedroom will become the center of Mom or Dad's universe. Just as you decorated the nursery with tender loving care, you should do the same with your dad's bedroom. However, you'll need to make sure that your dad doesn't become isolated and spend all of his time in the bedroom. Whenever physically possible, he needs to be out of bed and encouraged to be up and about. Make sure he gets dressed for the day and doesn't stay in bed clothes. A friend of mine had been a pharmacist who wore a suit every day to work. Even when he retired, he put on his suit. When he came down with Alzheimer's, his wife helped him put his suit on every day to give him a sense of respect and purpose.

Here are some bedroom decorating tips to make life easier for your mom or dad:

- If it's difficult for your dad to get in and out of bed, get a hospital bed. Medicare will usu-ally cover this cost but be sure to check ahead of time. It will also be much easier for you to provide care to your dad if, he is bedridden.

- If you can use a room that has a window, great. But your first priority is setting up a room near the bathroom. If this cannot be accomplished, then you'll need to get a portable commode. This, too, is often covered by Medicare.

- You can also rent healthcare equipment such as a table that swings across the bed for meals and other activities, a trapeze to help with heavy lifting, and a wheelchair.

- Set up a little visiting area with chairs and a small table so that family and friends can come to visit. It should also be an area where your mom can sit when she's able to get out of bed.

- Have a table next to the bed, so that your dad can easily reach for his glasses, his bottle of water, the telephone, the remote control for the television, and anything else that he frequently uses. But try not to clutter the table.

- Be sure to have a television and radio in the room that Mom can control.

- If your dad suffers from dementia, watch how he responds to wallpaper and pictures. If either seems to aggravate or confuse him (he tries to pick the flowers off flowered wallpaper or constantly pushes a circle thinking it will open something), replace it with soothing colors and quiet designs.

Senior Alert

Staying in bed can be dangerous to your parent's health, because the systems of the body get lazy and start to shut down. Muscles waste away; kidneys malfunction; blood pressure goes up; insulin production stops; fluid starts collecting in the lungs, leading to pneumonia; and blood clots start forming, increasing the possibility of an attack on the heart and brain.

- Give your mom the security of knowing that she can contact you while you're in another room in the house by using a room monitor (baby monitor) so she can call you without yelling. You might want to consider getting her a personal alert alarm.

- Get an egg-crate mattress pad for the bed to help prevent bed sores. It runs about $20 and you can get it at stores like K-mart, Wal-Mart, and Target. In fact, if your dad is coming from the hospital to live with you, chances are the hospital will give you one. But don't think the egg-crate pad will do the whole trick. You must also frequently reposition Dad (every few hours) to prevent bed sores. See Chapter 9, "A Trip to the Hospital," for more on bed sores.

- If your mom isn't giving medicines to herself, keep all the prescription bottles and medical supplies out of her sight. No one likes to be constantly reminded that she's "sick." Don't make the bedroom into a "sick room."

- Have a few plants and fresh flowers adorning the room. If your parent likes a chirping bird or singing canary and it doesn't pose a health hazard, take off to the pet shop. If you aren't bird people, there are always goldfish.

- Be sure to place a large clock and calendar in the room because it's very easy to get disoriented when you spend so much time in one room. If Dad has dementia, it's also helpful to have a magic marker board where you can write down things like what Dad has had for lunch, or what time you're coming back.

Whatever you do, keep the room clean with fresh bedding. We all know how good it feels to crawl between nice, clean sheets. That's one feeling that never fades away.

Nutrition—What's to Eat?

If you've ever had a hospital stay, you know how important mealtime becomes (unless you're relegated to Jell-O). With little else to do, you start to focus mostly on breakfast, lunch, and dinner. So don't be surprised if mealtime becomes all-important to your mom. Every morning, Grandma and I would have tea and toast. It became a ritual and a nice way for us to start the day. If I was running late, she'd start with, "Bread must be mighty scarce around here." That was my cue.

With today's hectic schedules and fast-food lifestyles, you might not have time for the regular sit-down meals that your parents had while they raised you. Yet, with the medications Mom is taking, it's better for her to be on a schedule. And it's always nicer if she doesn't have to eat alone. If you can't join Mom, set up a schedule of friends, neighbors, and relatives (even the grandkids) to enjoy one meal a day with her.

Besides the time and social aspect of eating, what your parent eats is *way* important, as my teens would say. For years now, we've been hearing, "you are what you eat."

(If so, my son's a taco and my daughter's a Biggie Fry.) And our parents … well they're the meat, potatoes, and gravy crowd. Whatever ethnic background they come from, chances are they like things heavy—heavy on sauces, salts, and spices. America's interest in low fat and light fare has been relatively recent. So it might take some doing to get Mom interested in foods that are user-friendly to her older body.

But if you're the one now preparing the meals, you have an edge. The researchers at Tuft's University Center on Nutrition played around with the USDA's Food Guide Pyramid and came up with a 70-plus pyramid, shown on the following page. Note two major differences: The base of the pyramid is water and the top has a flag recommending supplements in calcium, and vitamins D, and B-12. What's with the floating base? Dehydration is a major problem among the elderly. While Gen-Xers run around with trendy Evian bottles in hand, their grandparents are losing their sense of thirst. Before you know it the older set is having kidney problems, constipation, and other complications because the medications they take further deplete the body's water supply. Your dad may also be lowering his intake because getting to the bathroom is a hassle, your mom might cut down on water because she fears incontinence. Find out what underlies you parent's lack of water intake and correct it. Always keep a fresh glass handy, or get Dad to sport a younger look with his own water bottle.

You'll also notice on the 70-plus pyramid little f-pluses everywhere. These stand for fiber, and your parent needs plenty of it. Fiber is great stuff for the digestive track. And don't forget to salute the flag on top of the pyramid by giving your parent vitamin supplements.

Geri-Fact

According to AARP, four out of five older adults have chronic illnesses that are affected by diet; one out of eight suffers depression and loss of appetite; one in four drinks too much alcohol; one out of three lives alone and doesn't feel like cooking; and most take multiple medications that require a nutritionally sound body to be effective. Many older people are in a rut, eating the same thing day after day.

Here are a few other nutrition tips if you've now become your parent's chef:

- Talk with your parent's physician to see if your mom needs a special diet considering her illness. Ask to talk with a registered dietician to help you design a menu.

- Try serving small, frequent meals if your dad has lost his appetite. Or serve him the larger meal of the day when his appetite seems to peak.

- If your dad can't see very well, use plain white plates and lay out his food on the plate as if it were a clock. For example, tell him that the rice is at 9:00 o'clock, the chicken at noon, and the green beans at 4:00 o'clock.

- Make mealtime a special event with nice silverware, colorful napkins, and restaurant-like presentation of the food. When it comes to liquids, straws might make drinking easier.

- If your dad has trouble using utensils, try having finger foods on hand: vegetables and fruits that you've cut up, egg rolls, tea sandwiches, and good old chicken nuggets.

- If your mom suffers from dementia and keeps forgetting that she just ate, write out what she just had for lunch on a magic marker board. Have her repeat what she's eating while you write it on the board. Then put on the board what time she'll have her next meal.

- If you need to have meals brought in, don't forget to call your local area agency on aging to find out how to contact the closest Meals on Wheels program near you.

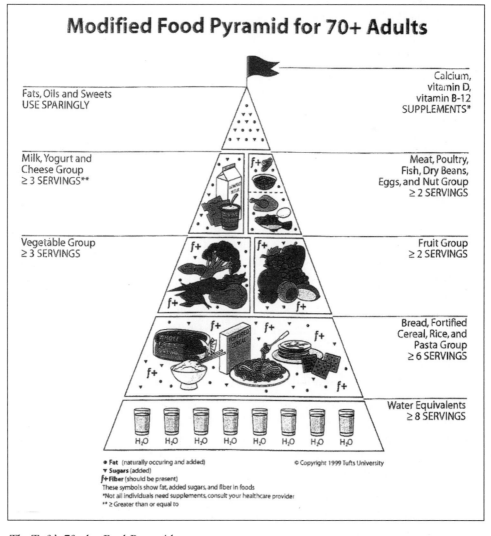

The Tuft's 70-plus Food Pyramid.

Sage Source

To track down handy utensils and ways to make eating easier, contact the Rehabilitation Center (1-800-346-2742) or Independent Living Aids (1-800-537-2118) and ask for catalogs on eating utensils and devices. Here are three terrific Web sites on nutrition:

- **The American Dietetic Association (www.eatright.org).** At this site you can search for a registered dietician near you for a consult.

- **The Tufts University Nutrition Navigator Nutritionists (www.navigator. tufts.edu).** This site reviews and rates a zillion Web sites on nutrition. You can hyperlink to those they review.

- **Mayo Clinic's Health Oasis (www.mayohealth.org/).** This site is fun and user-friendly, offering articles on nutrition, a virtual cookbook, and Ask a Dietician. You can even send in your favorite recipe for a "makeover" on how to make it less fattening and more healthy. Click on the Nutrition Center on the home page.

Bathing Strategies

Giving your parent a bath when they are either physically or mentally incapable of doing so themselves can be quite a challenge. If someone is suffering from dementia, taking a bath can be overwhelming: the barrage of water, removal of clothing, use of soap, fear of falling, and the feeling of privacy being invaded can create a wall of resistance. In their classic book *The 36-Hour Day* (see Appendix A, "Resources"), Nancy L. Mace and Peter V. Rabins suggest that you don't get into an argument over a bath. Instead you inform your dad of the basic steps and keep him moving along. So it's not, "Dad, you need to take a bath after breakfast," which only builds up anxiety. It's more like, "Dad, your bath water is ready." Then "Dad you need to unbutton your shirt." Even if he argues in between, keep focused on the next steps.

Bath water should be warm, never hot, because older skin is very fragile. Use very gentle soaps that are super-fatted or glycerin-based. Dry all areas, especially in skin folds, under the breasts, between the toes and genitals. Corn starch can provide added dryness in these areas. Apply nonperfumed lotion after the bath. While you're bathing your parent, be sure to check for rashes and any red spots that could flag an impending bedsore. Full baths or showers every day are not necessary for an older person and, in fact, could break down Mom or Dad's skin. On off days, a sponge bath will do. Be sure to invest in safety features for the bath and or shower to prevent falls. Any durable medical goods store can help you with these items and let you know what's covered under Medicare.

Caregiving and Dementia

None of us will ever know what it's like having Alzheimer's disease unless we go through it ourselves. If *Star Trek*'s Mr. Spock did one of his Vulcan mind-melds, he'd probably tell us that it feels like being lost—*all* of the time. Imagine the constant state of anxiety—not knowing anyone, never feeling like you're in familiar surroundings, never really being home. If that were your constant mental state, you can begin to appreciate why your dad might get panicky as soon as you leave, or get angry that he can't find his way back to his room or forgot how to button his shirt. You'll need to learn how to appreciate your dad's world so that the world you share together will be one of understanding and peace.

From my personal experience and what other experts in the field say, here's what we have learned in caring for someone with dementia (for more information, see Chapter 6, "Alzheimer's Disease and Cancer"):

- Try to develop a routine that you follow every day. You may be bored, but your dad will find the schedule comforting. Check off the day's schedule as you go along, so your dad can follow the day's events.

- To counter that "lost" feeling, label drawers, doors, and closets so Dad will know what's in them.

- Keep life simple! Your mom just can't handle a lot of input. It will frustrate her, and she may react in an outburst that will upset everyone around her. Don't act rushed or give her something to do that requires several steps at once. Break down tasks, one step at a time. For example, you don't

Sage Source

You can order *The 36-Hour Day* through Johns Hopkins University Press by calling 1-800-537-5487 or go to www.press.jhu.edu. It's also available at most bookstores. It's a must-read for anyone taking care of someone with Alzheimer's. Another book that's full of practical nursing care advice is *The Caregiver's Guide* by Caroline Rob, R.N. (see Appendix A).

Geri-Fact

Remember, if Mom has dementia, her behavior is not intentional. She is brain injured. Knowing this will help you handle your own emotions.

have to announce, "We're going to the doctor's in an hour," but rather, "Mom, let's put your coat on," "Let me help you to the door," "Mom, now we're going down the steps," "Here, we are at the car, let me get the door." If she wants to know where she's going, you could say that the doctor has been asking about her, and wouldn't it be nice to stop by and let him know how she's doing. In my situation, Grandma liked to visit. She didn't see the doctor's visit as threatening if I presented it to her this way. Think of the things your parent loved doing. Try to do things in that context.

- Take the time to observe your parent's new way of communicating to you. Watch for signs of what Mom does just before she becomes extremely agitated. Hopefully, you'll pick up a pattern so that you can remove or prevent what bothers her.

The Need to Wander

One of the greatest fears and challenges faced by many families is their parent's need to wander. Wandering is a frequent behavior among people with dementia. In fact, it is so common that many nursing homes have developed "wandering tracks" in their facilities, so that their wandering residents can safely wander when they feel the need. Now, chances are you don't have a wandering track at home, and if Mom does leave the house unattended, she poses safety risks for herself and others. Here are some tips to help you cope with her wandering:

- Get an ID bracelet with her name, your phone number, and "memory impaired" engraved on it. You can also purchase these through MedicAlert. You can visit their Web site at www.medicalert.com, or call 1-800-432-5378.

- Give your mom a card with your phone number on it, so she can call you if she is lost.

- Alert the local police and give them a photo of her, or contact any local store she would likely go to if she found a way out of your home.

- Install alarms that will set off if she's leaving the house, or use childproof devices to prevent her from opening an outside door.

- While you are with her, constantly reassure her where she is and that everything is fine.

- Find ways to get her to exercise or take her for walks. There are even exercises she can do while sitting in a chair.

Senior Alert

Be very careful of giving sedating medications or over-the-counter sleeping aids to someone who has dementia. Sometimes the drugs may have the opposite effect on a brain-injured person. Always check with the doctor before giving over-the-counter sleeping aids.

- Give your mom simple tasks to do during the day. If she loves folding clothes, bring out the towels every day to give her something to do.

- Reduce water intake several hours before bedtime, so she won't need to get up to urinate in the middle of the night risking a fall or inducing wandering.

- Get her involved in adult day care (see next chapter) to keep her active during the day and more likely to sleep at night and reduce the need to wander.

- Don't lock Mom in a room or tie her in bed thinking that you're trying to keep her from hurting herself—she will, anyway. Besides, restraining her in this fashion is psychologically abusive.

- Observe what she does before she begins to wander, and see if you can identify a pattern. Look for the cause and make the changes accordingly.

The Least You Need to Know

- Take the time to accident-proof the house and create a bedroom that doesn't appear like a "sick room" and is near a bathroom.

- Turn into a geriatric-friendly chef and follow the 70-plus Food Pyramid Guidelines—lots of water, fiber, and vitamin supplements.

- Caring for someone with dementia is tough work; remember, that person is brain injured, and unpleasant behavior isn't intentional. Learn what to do.

- Bathing can be an overwhelming experience for someone with dementia. Be sensitive to Mom or Dad's needs to make it a safe and relaxing experience.

- People with Alzheimer's disease are prone to wander. You can add safety features to your home to alert you if your parent has opened a door to the outside. Giving Mom or Dad exercises and activities also will lessen the need to wander.

Chapter 19

You Can't Do It All

In This Chapter

- Understanding your emotions about caregiving
- Don't go it alone: getting help
- The benefits of adult day services and respite services
- Taking time for your spouse
- When to let go
- A creed for all caregivers

Of all the things I've ever done, taking care of Grandma during her last (and ninety-sixth) year of life was the toughest, most moving and deeply fulfilling of all. Would I do it again? In a heart beat. And yet, there did come a time when I had to let go, when I had to realize that caring for her was beyond my capacity. If you're caring for your parent now, or think you may down the line, remember one thing: You must take care of yourself!

If you've ever flown, you've heard the flight attendant give the direction "in case we lose cabin pressure" to put that dangling oxygen mask on *you* first—and then your child. Now there's a directive that goes against your maternal instincts. But if you're out of breath, you won't be in a position to help your child. In the same way, you need to take care of yourself before you can find the energy to take care of an aging parent, and that's the subject of this chapter.

What You May Feel About Caregiving

Each of us reacts differently to any situation. And so it is with caregiving. Be prepared to experience a wide range of emotions, from anger, guilt, sadness, and frustration to fulfillment, joy, and compassion. Some days will be like a rollercoaster, your emotions thrusting you from high to low in no time at all. You'll have these feelings toward not only your parent, but also other family members. So many caregivers report that they become frustrated with the lack of understanding and support from other family members, especially siblings. Just know that it is normal for you to experience such a wide range of emotions. The goal, however, is to achieve some balance and home in on the emotions that are healthy for you.

Walking in somebody else's shoes always gives you a better appreciation of what someone's going though and why that person behaves the way he or she does. Suffering from a chronic, debilitating condition has both physical and mental consequences. The more you understand the nature of your dad's condition(s) and how this affects his emotional well-being can take the sting out of his anger or frustration that he displaces on you.

Geri-Fact

The National Family Caregivers Association's national profile of caregivers found that 67 percent of caregivers felt frustration while nearly 40 percent felt sad and anxious. Half of all caregivers experienced back pain, sleeplessness, and depression.

Knowing the different stages of Alzheimer's, the clinical signs of depression, or the behavioral complications of Parkinson's will give you a heads-up on why Dad acts the way he does. It also reassures you that this isn't personal. The parent-child relationship is often wrought with unresolved conflicts. So, if you don't understand what's really going on, your dad's offensive behavior can open an old wound. There you are—tired, stressed-out, feeling unappreciated—and here he is hurting you, just like years past. Bang. Now you're angry. You react. He picks up on your agitation and things quickly spiral out of control. You need help in dealing with the situation.

Getting Help

I love those disclaimers after *Superman* that tell kids "don't try this at home." There should be a similar disclaimer that comes with caring for aging parents: "Don't do this alone." You'll be surprised at how quickly you can become isolated from family and friends. You'll start to feel that it's easier to just do things yourself. Or your parent will become so dependent upon you, that he or she never wants you to leave.

Grandma called me her "manager." She'd tell the doctors, the adult day care staff, and her adult grandchildren that they would have to go through her manager. We all thought it was pretty endearing, but she also reached a point where no one else but her manager could take care of her. This became especially tough when my baby was born. For a while, I tried to do it all. But caring friends pulled me aside to help me get some balance. I brought in a nurse's aide to help during the day. The few times I did go out when the baby got older, I had to bring in two separate caretakers. Many caregivers will tell you that they give up trying to go out and "have a life" because it's too much of a hassle getting help.

So before you find yourself caught up in a vicious cycle, search for help right away and set up a support system. Your parent can survive a few hours and even days without you. Let's look at some of the ways you can enlist help.

Join a Support Group

One way to get help is to join a support group. Other caregivers can share with you what they're going through and how they manage to cope. There's nothing like advice from those who have *been there*. Just about every disease has support groups that have professionals who provide solid, technical information about the disease and steps you can take to treat the condition. If your parent suffers from dementia, I can't recommend highly enough that you join an Alzheimer's support group. If joining a group isn't for you (at least give it a try), take advantage of the Internet and do your research on your parent's disease and join a chat room or discussion board of other caregivers.

Here are some tips on finding a support group:

- Most local hospitals offer community education programs and host support groups. Call the hospital's public affairs office to find out their offerings and schedule.

- Under Associations in the Yellow Pages you'll find the names of organizations that are dedicated to a particular disease, such as the Heart Association, Diabetic Association, Cancer Society, Stroke Association. Give them a call to track down a support group.

- Contact the National Alzheimer's Association (1-800-272-3900) to find a chapter located near you.

- Call Children of Aging Parents (1-800-227-7294) for information and referral services.

Sage Source

The following caregiver Web sites provide great information, as well as host chat rooms and discussion boards: www.caregiver.com, www.caregiving.com, and www.caregiving.org.

Involve Other Family Members

Usually, in the beginning, family members will be gung-ho on helping out. But then as time wears on everyone gets too busy. So, involve them early and set up the expectation that this is a family affair even though Dad is living with you. Give out-of-town family members tasks, such as tracking down medical information on the Internet, making calls to set up appointments, or shopping around for medical equipment. I highly recommend using e-mail—the family can be on a group list, and you can give weekly updates on what needs to be done and how Dad is doing. Someone can handle insurance matters or find community services that can assist you, another can order supplies and durable medical goods. Ask family members to identify blocks of time when they would like to visit Dad. Explain to them that you would like to use this time for you to get away. Even if it's a day trip, it's important for you to be away from your caregiving responsibilities. If you have family who live in the same area, then set up a weekly schedule of when they'll come to visit to relieve you.

Take Advantage of Community Services

Many area agencies on aging offer family caregiving support programs that can assist you in caring for your parent. Call the Eldercare Locator (1-800-677-1116) to find out if your local agency has such programs. If you work and find it difficult to handle meal preparation, call the local Meals on Wheels office. If this option doesn't work, there are many new catering businesses sprouting up to meet the needs of the baby boomer generation on the go.

Whenever a friend or family member says, "Gee, I wish I could help," rather than simply thank someone for the offer, take that person up on it! How about responding with, "You know what would be a great help … making Dad dinner some night next week." Or, "If you'd like to sit with him for a few hours, it would give me a chance to get out." Most people simply don't know what to do, and they'll appreciate the suggestion.

Whenever someone wants to give you a gift, think of things that make your life less stressful, such as being treated to a housecleaning service or even a massage. The A Quick Look At Community Services table in Chapter 12, "Living in the Community: Services and Transportation," gives you lots of ideas of the services available to you. Take the time up front to make these arrangements—it will be well worth the effort.

Sage Source

A wonderful book that can help you through the challenges of caregiving is by former First Lady Rosalynn Carter, *Helping Yourself Help Others* (see Appendix A, "Resources"). It's a warm, easy read, inspiring, and full of resources and practical advice.

Hire Help

The other avenue to get help, of course, is to hire it. Be sure to go over Chapter 10, "Home Health Care," for information on hiring help that's appropriate for your mom's level of care. If your siblings are wondering what they can do to help out (or need to be given a hint), get them to pitch in for home health care. Perhaps giving your dad a bath is downright dangerous for you—he's paralyzed on one side and is overweight. It might make sense to have a professionally trained person come in once a week and assist with the bath. If your parent constantly keeps you up all night, it might make sense to have someone come in to cope with his night wanderings so that you can get some sleep. Sleep deprivation is something that most caregivers experience, and it places them at great risk for physical problems themselves. I remember all too well my own exhaustion; I had just gotten the baby to sleep through the night when Grandma started to stay up through the night. And she wanted to be with me. After a few weeks of this, we hired night help. But as you can imagine, this became pretty expensive.

Be sure to check with your local area agency on aging to learn of any programs available to help you with homemaker services, chore services, and home health care. Ask your parent's physician if he or she knows of any services to assist you in your caregiving. Let the doctor know what you are dealing with at home and see what home health care he or she can prescribe.

Silver Lining

Rather than focus on your parent, identify the things that would make *your* life simpler. Would a taxi service make it easier to transport Mom to and from the doctor so you don't have to deal with the hassle of parking? How about a cleaning service coming in once a week? Find a pharmacist who delivers, so you're not running out to get prescriptions. Or find a grocery store that delivers—many are taking orders from the Internet these days. Get your hair done, have your nails manicured, get a massage, go out to lunch, see a movie—whatever makes your life better must be a priority. It's oxygen!

Adult Day Services to the Rescue

When I took in Grandma, I was working at an adult day services center. She loved the idea that she was going to work with me. She also fell in love with the program,

Geri-Fact

Medicare does not cover adult day services. Most people pay for the service out of pocket, which averages around $35 per day—quite a bargain, considering the cost to hire someone to just sit with your parent all day. Some Medicaid programs cover adult day care and many area agencies on aging subsidize the cost to make it reasonable. Call the local AAA (1-800-677-1116) to find out about programs in your area.

Sage Source

To find an adult day services program near you, call the National Adult Day Services Association at 202-479-0735 or visit their Web site at www.ncoa.org/nadsa and ask for a directory of adult day programs by city and state.

and there was a marked improvement in her mental health. It also allowed me to pursue my work and spend time with the baby. Adult day services (also known as adult day care) programs are all-day, supervised programs for older people who suffer from chronic conditions, often dementia. One thing all participants have in common is that they cannot be safely left alone. Most adult day service centers offer transportation services and a range of program activities for their participants. Most centers offer memory therapy, exercise programs, speech and music therapy, and other activities that help with your parent's mental and physical functioning. The centers provide emotional support to families and can teach them caregiving basics. Families who use adult day services often rave about it. Without it, many feel they wouldn't have been able to care for their parent at home. Today, most caregivers work, so caring for a parent at home would be out of the question if they didn't have these services to depend on.

Look for a program that has a nurse and social worker highly involved in the program. Ask about staff training, and ask what the staff/client ratio is: Depending on the care needs of the clients, there should be at least one worker for every six people. Also ask to see their activity schedule. Hang in there with your parent—it may take a few times to get Mom used to it. Many families have found it helpful to introduce the idea of going to adult day services as something Mom has always loved doing: She's going there to play cards, to volunteer, or to have a day out with the "girls."

Respite Care

Respite care can come in many shapes and sizes. The focus is on you. It's about you getting a break (respite) from your caregiving—in other words, getting more oxygen. Some people use adult day services as respite care, using it two or three days a week. Others bring in family members to get away for the day. Find a way to get consistent breaks in your caregiving. If you have not had a vacation for far too long and your spouse is begging to go or you want to make your niece's wedding, then contact a local nursing home or assisted living facility. Many of them have rooms available for short stays (less than a month) so that you can leave knowing your parent is being well cared for.

The National Senior Corps will send trained volunteers to your home once a week to be a companion to your parent so that you can get some respite. Call their hotline (1-800-424-8867) for the number of the program closest to you. Many churches and synagogues offer volunteers that provide family caregivers respite care as part of a national "interfaith volunteer caregivers" program. Go through your Yellow Pages and call faith-based organizations to see if they offer such a service.

Support Your Spouse

The profile of the average caregiver is a woman in her late 50s or early 60s who holds a job and is married. Even if you're married to the greatest guy on Earth with the patience of Job, caring for your parent (or his) will test your marriage. If you're the spouse of a caregiver reading this, please look out for your partner. Know that your partner is trying the best she can, and that she probably has mixed feelings about caregiving. Your partner probably feels pulled in all directions and is also concerned that she's not paying enough attention to you. Get your spouse to go to support groups by going along with her or offering to watch Dad while she goes. Both of you need to understand the medical conditions you are dealing with. Don't ignite a fiery exchange between your spouse and her mom. Become a calming influence.

And for those of you providing the care, don't forget to take time out to be with your spouse. Remember the days when you were raising your kids and what you'd go through to have a night out. Well, those days are back. Don't let caregiving consume your entire life. Try not to have serious, heavy discussions before going to bed. Schedule a separate time to discuss caregiving issues. View it as a project that you and your spouse are *both* working on, as in *we're in the same boat*. Communicate your needs to each other, and don't assume that you know how the other feels. Your husband might be building up feelings of resentment because he's afraid bringing up something that's bothering him will send you over the top. Communicate. Communicate. And make the time to enjoy each other!

Knowing When to Let Go

You may be blessed to have a caregiving situation where you're able to manage your family life and care for your mom or dad until his or her death. If you are able to pull together a support system that nurtures both you and your parent, you'll long remember these days as having given your mom a gift. You may, however, have done all of this and then reach a point when you physically and mentally cannot provide

Senior Alert

If you're reaching a point where you feel yourself "going down"—you've become isolated from family and friends, you've been sick, your children feel estranged from you, you're feeling depressed, anxious and pulled in all directions—it's time to re-think your decision to be a caregiver. Call a family meeting and talk to a professional to help you assess the situation. You've got to seek help.

Sage Source

If you are a spiritual person, you might appreciate the solace from this book, *Caregiving, the Spiritual Journey of Love, Loss and Renewal* by Beth Witrogen McLeod (see Appendix A). The author shares her own experience and how you can find strength through religion and spirituality.

the level of care your parent needs. In fact, in some instances, it may not be safe for you to provide the care, and you'll be causing more harm than good.

Sometimes, your family doctor or another health care professional can help you see more clearly what you need to do. There are some excellent nursing homes that can provide top-flight care in a very dignified way. Chapter 15, "Choosing a Nursing Home," provides you with the guidance to find a good home. Many people are living much longer these days with complicated conditions that require sophisticated care that may simply be beyond your capabilities. These actually become the easier, less guilt-ridden decisions. The tough decisions often center on cost when you can't afford the home care that your parent demands. 'Round-the-clock care can get very expensive, even if the care your parent needs is provided by those who make just above the minimum wage (for example, a companion service).

I had hoped to keep Grandma with us until the end. However, she began to have ministrokes, and we had to invest in round-the-clock care which was running us $80 a day (18 years ago). She had also become very combative, paranoid, and incontinent. Even as I write this, I still feel some guilt and the need to justify letting her go. Yet, I know it was for the best for her and us. The home we placed her in was excellent and within just a few miles. I was able to visit her every few days with the baby. And I was with her the day she died reciting her favorite psalm.

It's never easy making these kinds of life choices. There's plenty of *could haves, would haves,* and *ifs* in life. Stick with what *is* and what you need to do. If your motives are in the best interest of both of you—you'll do just fine.

Caregiver's Creed

Most caregivers are pretty generous souls—that's why they've taken on this assignment in the first place. So it may take some doing to convince them that they do have rights and need to set some limits on the extent they'll go to take care of someone they love. Here's a creed for caregivers:

- Ask for help. Let other know what you need.
- Empower yourself through knowledge, understand your parent's condition.
- Set limits on what you will do and let others know.
- Take care of your physical and mental health.
- Take regular breaks from caregiving.
- Keep up your interests and hobbies.
- Know that you have a right to a life of your own.
- Forgive yourself; it's okay to be angry and resentful at times. Don't dwell on your shortcomings; move on.
- Laugh. And laugh some more!
- Don't burn out your spouse—nurture your marriage.
- Take control, create a support network to help you with your caregiving tasks.
- Take joy in the good you are doing.

The Least You Need to Know

- One of the best ways to get a handle on your emotions is to understand the behavioral effects of your parent's disease or condition.
- Caregiving is not a solo act—get control by setting up a support system to help you care for your parent.
- You must take breaks. Arrange for respite care and take a look at adult day services for your parent, especially if you work.
- You have the right to take care of yourself, laugh, keep up your interests, forgive yourself, and not allow your caregiving to consume you.
- There may come a time when nursing home care is the best thing for your parent. It's okay to let the home take care of your parent when their medical needs are beyond your capabilities.

Chapter 20

End-of-Life Matters
and Hospice

In This Chapter

- What is important to dying people
- How to talk about end-of-life decisions
- The five stages of coming to terms with dying
- The hospice alternative
- The value of good family communication

If you've been taking care of your parent at home and are able to do so up to Mom or Dad's death, you will have given your parent and yourself a very special gift. The operative words are *able to do so*. Not everyone is either emotionally or physically up for this kind of care. In fact, your parent's condition may warrant care that can be provided only outside of the home.

Whether or not you plan to care for your parent while he or she is dying, this chapter will help you understand the decisions you need to consider and the options available. Hopefully, it will also help you cope with one of life's most heart-wrenching milestones, letting go of your parents.

What Most People Want When They're Dying

In a recent comprehensive study conducted by the Veterans Affairs Medical Center in Durham, North Carolina, researchers interviewed terminally ill patients, their doctors, social workers, hospice volunteers, chaplains, and family members. The researchers found six elements that are integral to creating a positive end-of-life experience:

- Preventing pain was the most important to patients. Many people feared dying in pain more than dying itself. Doctors can be very helpful, managing pain and reassuring both patients and their families that pain can be controlled.

- Patients want to be involved in making decisions regarding their treatment. Gone are the hush-hush days of "saving" the patient from the truth. Letting the patient's desires direct decision-making relieves families of guilt should the patient desire less treatment, and prevents conflicts and debates among family members. What Mom or Dad wants becomes the unifying rallying point.

- Patients and families need to know what to expect from the fatal condition and the treatment. This knowledge helps them better prepare for events, symptoms, and treatment outcomes surrounding the impending death.

- Patients and families search for meaningfulness to their lives and their relationship with each other at the end of life. They'll seek the solace of faith, review their lives, resolve conflicts, spend time with family and friends, and say goodbye.

- Patients find satisfaction in contributing to he well-being of others. They find peace in helping their loved ones come to terms with their dying and helping loved ones let go. They also find it satisfying to leave behind the means to care for their loved one's physical and financial needs.

- Patients do not want to be seen as a "disease" or a "case," but as a unique, whole person.

Geri-Fact

The dying process has been extended in American society due to medical technology and the management of pneumonia, renal failure, and other infections. Nearly three out of every four people who die in America are 65 years and older. Most die in hospitals or nursing homes. As a result, many adults never experience living with or caring for someone who is dying.

From this research and many other similar studies, it is clear that honest, compassionate communication—no matter how painful the topic—is crucial to a "good death."

Finding the Words

We live in a society of euphemisms. Rather than saying someone has died, we say "passed on." Rather than say, hundreds of people are losing their jobs, we say the company was "downsized." So how do you have a straightforward conversation about dying with your mom or dad? Do you really need to even have the conversation? If we're to listen to the researchers and all of those who have "been there," the answer is yes.

It's not uncommon for those who are dying to give you cues and opportunities to engage in the conversation. It might start off with a vague reference of *when I'm gone* or *let's go over my finances* or they might start giving you things that were mutually understood to be given to you after their death. Don't walk away from these moments. Your instinct might be to say, "Come on, Mom, you're fine," or "Let's talk about it another time." If your parent brings it up, engage the opportunity.

Share with your parent how hard the conversation is for you, too. How much he or she means to you and how you can't imagine being without Mom or Dad. But also share with your parent how much you want to treasure this final time together, and that means carefully planning and making decisions now so that Mom or Dad's needs can be met.

If, on the other hand, your parent hasn't brought it up, you might need to be the one to do so. The National Hospice Foundation recently commissioned a study on American opinions about end-of-life decisions. They learned that one out of four baby boomers would not bring up issues related to their parent's death even if they knew their parent had only six months to live. Yet, parents said that they would rely on family members to carry out their wishes. Now, wait a minute. How are you going to know those wishes without talking about it?

Here are some suggestions from the National Hospice Foundation (and some thoughts from my own experience) on how to talk with Mom and Dad regarding end-of-life decisions:

- Before initiating the discussion, do some homework and learn about the end-of-life options in your community (hospice care, volunteers, home health services, faith-based programs). Plan for the discussion; it's really not a spur of the moment kind of thing.

- Familiarize yourself with advance directives, living wills, durable power of attorney, and "Do Not Resuscitate" orders (see Chapters 24, "Planning for Incapacity," and 25, "Lawyers, Wills, and Estate Planning"). Doing so will help you determine the kinds of questions you need to explore with your parent, so you'll have the answers.

- Choose a quiet, private place to hold a one-on-one conversation.

- Ask permission from your parent to have the discussion. For example, "Dad, I'd like to talk about how you would like to be cared for if you got really sick. Is that okay?" Or, "Mom, I really want to do the right thing if you ever got very sick. I'd feel better if I knew what you want. Could we talk about it?"

- Allow your parent to set the pace. Don't rush in to fill up the silence. Stay focused: You are having this conversation because you want to learn from your parent what his or her wishes are so that you can fulfill *Mom or Dad's* needs. This isn't about you.

- Listen. Repeat what you've heard your parent say to you. For example, "Mom, what I hear you say is that you want to stay at home for as long as possible. In fact, if it's medically possible and you won't be in pain, you would rather spend your last days here at home rather than in the hospital."

- Once you've had this discussion, you can set up another time to detail Mom or Dad's wishes in writing through an advance directive or a living will (see Chapter 24).

Remember, the goal of this discussion is to help you find out what your mom or dad wants regarding his or her end-of-life care. Your job is to assure Mom or Dad that his or her needs and wishes will be met.

Some people won't discuss the issue no matter what, and you'll need to respect your parent's wishes. Or you, personally, might find it an impossible task. Perhaps someone else in the family is better suited to have the conversation.

Coming to Terms with Dying

When you and your dad come to the realization that his condition is terminal, there are a number of stages each of you may go through. Chances are you will not go through these stages in sync with each other. Dr. Elisabeth Kübler-Ross wrote a now famous book, *On Death and Dying* (see Appendix A) in the late 1960s, which broke new ground in our understanding of how people cope with dying and death. Through interviews and counseling of terminally ill patients, Dr. Ku[um]bler-Ross shared the following observations of five basic stages many people go through as they come to terms with dying:

1. **Denial.** At first, you simply can't believe it is true. The realization that life will end—even if you have lived a long life—is too much to absorb. Denial is the mind's shock absorber, giving you a chance to soak in the reality of dying. So if you and your Dad act like nothing has really changed, it's okay. At least for a while.

2. **Anger.** If you're on the receiving end of your dad's anger, you might think this isn't such a great stage. However, anger means that your dad is past denying his condition. He may be angry at his physician, the nurses trying to care for him, God, family members, friends, or he may be just angry at life itself. Let him express his anger. He'll need to go through this before he can move on to acceptance.

3. **Bargaining.** Ever secretly make a deal with God—or whatever higher power you believe in—that if you do a certain good thing, then you'll get something in return. Or you'll look for a "sign" to help you make a big decision? That's what the bargaining stage is essentially all about. Your parent may be bargaining for more time. Perhaps, your mom wants to hold on until a special family event—a reunion, a wedding, or birth of a grandchild. During this period, you may see your mom becoming very active in her health care trying to gain control. If you see this in your mom, explore what her hopes are and assist her in making it happen.

4. **Depression.** Once it becomes undeniably clear that all the bargaining in the world won't change the inevitable, your dad will likely become depressed. He'll be mourning the loss of his life, of the things to come and the things he didn't get to do. During this period it is helpful to thank your parent for all that he or she has done for you. Acknowledge what Dad has accomplished during his lifetime. He'll need this time to mourn and will probably do so, quietly and in private. Antidepressants and cheery conversation won't make it go away. Nor should it. It's a healthy response to the realization that his life is ending.

5. **Acceptance.** Hopefully, your parent will reach this final stage, when he or she peacefully accepts the fact that death is near. Mom will begin to disengage—she may tell you that she doesn't want any more visitors. She will not want to go through the emotional hard work of repeated good-byes. Chances are you aren't going to reach this stage at the same time as your parent. You, or perhaps one of your siblings, might be angry and want Mom to fight this by trying a new treatment therapy to buy more time. You'll need to respect where she is. Don't push her back after she's finally come to terms with dying.

Perhaps being aware of the various stages that many people experience in response to the dying of a loved one may help you better understand your own feelings and those of your siblings and surviving parent. Each of you will handle your feelings differently; just stay focused on what your dying parent needs and most of the rest will fall into place.

Sage Source

There are two excellent Web sites that provide an extensive list of books and links to other sites on dying and death. At Dr. Ira Byock's Web site (www.dyingwell.org) you'll find that each book is linked to Amazon.com so that you can get a synopsis of the book. The award-winning Growth House site (www.growthhouse.org) brings together just about everything you need to know on dying and death. It also offers synopses of the books they recommend. Bookmark these sites!

What Is Hospice?

Hospice care involves a team approach bringing together medical care, pain management, and emotional and spiritual support to patients and their families. This care is provided in either the patient's home or a home-like setting of an inpatient hospice facility. Those who receive hospice care are at the advanced stages of their disease. The mission of hospice staff and volunteers is to address the symptoms of an illness with the intent of promoting comfort and dignity. They are experts at pain management.

Geri-Fact

According to the American Hospice Foundation, **hospice** is "comprehensive care in the last months of life. Hospice services are provided by a team of doctors, nurses, social workers, grief and spiritual counselors, physical therapists, home health aides, and volunteers. Wherever possible, care is provided at home." But when it can't be, hospice care is provided at a home-like inpatient facility.

Many people are of the misconception that hospice is a place where people with cancer go to die. First of all, about 80 percent of hospice care is provided in the home. And secondly, although many of the people they care for are dying of cancer, they also help those dying of the end stages of chronic diseases like heart disease, emphysema, and Alzheimer's. Hospice provides care for all ages.

Based upon my personal experience with hospice and my professional work training hospice volunteers, I can't reinforce enough to you how helpful hospice can be to you and your family. Hospice can manage your parent's pain, help you understand what your mom or dad is going through, and help you cope with your own emotions. Although death is a natural part of life, it still remains a mystery. We are often at a loss regarding what we should do before and at the time of death. The hospice folks can get you through it at your own pace. They also stay in touch with you following your loved one's death.

When to Call for Hospice

Hospice care is meant to help your parent (and the family) through the last stages of an illness. The eligibility rules of Medicare set definite parameters of when to seek hospice care. A physician and the hospice medical director must confirm that your parent has a life expectancy of less than six months. Your parent must also agree that he or she will not pursue treatments for curing the terminal illness.

So, if your mom is aware of her terminal illness, she's decided that she's not going to seek any life-extending procedures, and she would like to die at home, then hospice is an excellent option for her. If you decide that you want to give a dying-at-home experience for her, then I'd highly recommend calling in hospice to help you with the care and respite that you'll surely need. Be sure to work with your mom's family doctor on this decision. The doctor is the one to make the referral. Hospice care will also save you and your family from financial hardship.

Sage Source

I recommend the following Web sites on hospice care: Hospice Foundation of America (www.hospicefoundation.org), 1-800-854-3402; National Hospice and Palliative Care Organization (www.nhpco.org), 703-243-5900; and American Hospice Foundation (www.americanhospice.org), 202-223-0204.

Medicare Covers Hospice Care

Many people don't realize it but Medicare offers a hospice benefit that will cover almost all of the costs of caring for a dying person during his or her last six months of life. To qualify for the Medicare hospice benefit …

- Your parent must have Medicare Part A.
- Your doctor and the medical director of the hospice must confirm that your parent has a life expectancy of less than six months.
- Your parent must agree in writing that he or she will not pursue any treatments to cure his or her illness.

As a Medicare beneficiary, your parent can choose any Medicare-certified hospice in your area. Even if your parent belongs to a Medicare managed care plan, your parent has this benefit. You do not have to be pre-certified nor do you have to use a hospice in the HMO's network. Nor does your parent need to get out of the managed care plan. If your parent needs services from the managed care plan, beyond hospice care, it will be covered as long as your parent remains enrolled.

The Medicare hospice benefit covers the following:

- Skilled nursing services
- Volunteer services
- Physician visits
- Skilled therapy
- Medical social services
- Spiritual counseling
- Nutrition counseling
- Bereavement support for the family

The benefit also covers 95 percent of the cost of prescription drugs for symptom control and pain relief, short-term inpatient respite care to relieve family members from caregiving, and home care. Most hospices cover the remaining 5 percent of the cost. Equipment is also covered. The Medicare hospice benefit does not cover 24-hour care in the home; however, in a medical crisis, continuous nursing and short-term inpatient services are available.

Geri-Fact

Many hospice organizations are now adding the word "palliative" to their names. Palliative care seeks to address not only physical pain but also emotional, social, and spiritual pain to achieve the best quality of life for patients and their families.

If no one can take care of your parent at home, hospice care is available in some nursing homes and hospitals. And there are also some programs available that can help place home health care workers in the home. Be aware, however, that Medicare does not pay for full-time home health care.

The hospice team is available 24 hours a day to those patients being cared for at home to respond to any possible emergencies. They'll provide medications, home visits, and arrange for other care as needed and reimbursed by Medicare. The day-to-day, 'round-the- clock care, however, is provided by a complement of family, friends, and home health aides covered by insurance or private pay.

Finding a Hospice

Whatever hospice you decide upon, be sure that it is a Medicare-certified facility. These are the only hospice programs that are eligible to receive your parent's Medicare Hospice Benefit. There are over 2,400 hospice programs throughout the country. Three good sources of information regarding hospice programs available in your community are the local area agency on aging, your local hospital's department of social services, and your regional home health intermediary (RHHI). And of course, there's always the trusted Yellow Pages of your phone book.

Sage Source

Visit Medicare's Web site (www.medicare.gov) and click on "Important Contacts," where you can find the phone number of the regional home health intermediary. Give them a call and they'll tell you how to contact the Medicare-certified hospices in your area. You can also call Medicare at 1-800-633-4277. Or visit the National Hospice Organization Web site (www.nhpco.org); you can click on a map that will give you a list of hospices in your area.

Questions to Ask a Hospice Provider

Your parent's primary physician should be a good resource in referring you to a hospice. Ask the doctor if he or she has a working relationship with any particular hospice and if it is positive. Here are some questions to ask when inquiring about a hospice:

- Is the hospice Medicare-certified?
- Is the hospice a member of any professional organization or has it been accredited?
- Are there certain conditions that patients and families have to meet to enter the hospice program?
- Would the hospice be willing to come to the home and conduct an assessment to help you and your parent decide that this is the best option?
- What specialized services does the hospice offer (rehabilitation therapists, family counselors, pharmacists, used equipment)?
- What are the hospice's policies regarding inpatient care? What hospitals does it have contractual relationships with in the event your parent would need to go to the hospital?
- Does the hospice require a primary family caregiver as a condition of admission? What are the caregiver's responsibilities as related to the hospice?
- What kind of emergency coverage does it offer? Who is on call? Will a nurse come quickly to the home, if needed?
- What out-of-pocket expenses can we expect?
- Will the hospice handle all of the paperwork and billing?

- What are the hospice's policies on the use of antibiotics, ventilators, dialysis, enteral or parenteral nutrition (nutrients given intravenously)? What treatments does it consider outside its purview?

Some Parting Words About Family

Years ago, I spent a year working as a nursing assistant and counselor in an emergency room and intensive care unit. Other than giving the nurses an extra hand, my major job was to act as the nursing staff's liaison with families who had a loved one who was in critical condition or had just died. As families would anxiously wait for news about their loved one's condition, I would sit with them. Other times, I'd go back and forth between the medical staff and families, updating them on any progress being made. The toughest times of all were gathering the family in a private room so that the doctor could tell them that someone they cherished "didn't make it." It's a year that's never left me.

What I learned from being with family members in such times of need is that those who had a good history of being able to communicate as a *family* fared much better than those who didn't. All too often, a son who hadn't talked to his dad for months, or even years, stood there with total regret that he couldn't patch things up. Brothers and sisters who hadn't resolved old conflicts fought all the more when it came to making major end-of-life decisions regarding their parent. These decisions are deeply personal, calling up strong emotions as to how we view our *own* death. Even siblings who get along fairly well can find themselves in a highly charged debate over what is in Mom's best interest.

The best way that parents can preserve family unity is to decide for themselves what is in their best interest. Perhaps, if they approach grappling with an advance directive as a way of preventing a wedge or conflict among their children after they're gone, they'll see the task for what it really is: an act of love.

And the greatest lesson I learned from that year? Never let an argument go unresolved between you and a loved one past bed time. Never storm out of the house and jump in a car in a fit of anger. Too much of the death that I saw stole from people the moment they had all planned on—to make up. You simply never know.

Sage Source

Some other sites of interest include Death with Dignity National Center (www.deathwithdignity. org), 202-530-2900; Americans for Better Care of the Dying (www. absd-caring. org); and Last Acts (lastacts.rwjf.org).

The Least You Need to Know

- Two of the most important things people want when they are dying is to control the pain and control the decisions regarding their treatment.

- Families do much better if they know what their parent's wishes are in *advance* as to end-of-life decisions. Advance directives prevent family conflict.

- Most people come to terms with dying in five stages: denial, anger, bargaining, depression, and acceptance.

- Hospice care is primarily provided in the home, or in a home-like setting of an inpatient hospice facility.

- Medicare provides every beneficiary a hospice benefit that covers nearly all costs during the last six months of life (even prescriptions) if your parent uses hospice care.

- In times of need, those who have a good history of being able to communicate as a family fare much better than those who don't.

Part 5
Financial and Legal Matters

How do you hold on to your money with the costs of long-term care pounding at your door? First you need to understand the basics of the "M&Ms": Medicare, the federal health insurance program; and Medicaid, the state program. Once you get some footing on this front, you'll discover the benefits your parents may be entitled to from organizations like the Department of Veterans Affairs.

Then it's on to beating daily out-of-pocket expenses and deciding whether or not long-term care insurance is a smart bet for your parents. And, last but not least, we enter the world of elder law: how to plan for incapacity, living wills, power of attorney, wills, trusts, and being an executor. We give you tips on how to find an elder law lawyer. For those of you who feel a little nervous about approaching your parents on the topic of what they plan on leaving behind, we share some advice on having the conversation.

Chapter 21

Got to Have Those M&Ms: Medicare and Medicaid

In This Chapter

- How Medicare works
- Bridging the gap with Medi-gap
- What Medicare covers—and what it doesn't
- The difference between original Medicare and Medicare managed care
- Doctors who take what Medicare assigns
- The difference between Medicare and Medicaid

Medicaid and Medicare. They sure sound alike, but they are quite different. Between the two, these guys pick up the tab for most of the care for the elderly in the whole country. One pays for almost all of the hospital care no matter what your income. The other pays for nursing home care, but it *does* matter what your income is—and it must be low.

There's plenty of misinformation going around that can put you in financial ruin. So let's get you up to speed. But know that just like speed limits, the rules can change. Our information is based on Medicare rules as of January 2000. Keep current by visiting Medicare's excellent Web site at www.medicare.gov.

Medicare: What Is It?

Medicare is a federal health insurance program. It is for three groups of people:

- People 65 years of age and over
- Some disabled people under the age of 65 years
- People with end-stage renal disease (folks with permanent kidney failure who are using dialysis or have had a kidney transplant)

Everyone receiving Social Security at age 65 automatically gets a Medicare card. If your parents aren't getting Social Security at that age, then they need to apply for it through their Social Security office. There are specific enrollment periods—so don't wait. Dad can apply three months before he turns 65 years old and up to four months after. If he misses the window, Dad could be in for some real hassles and a penalty.

There are two parts to Medicare:

1. **Part A.** This part is *not* optional. (Nor would you want it to be.) Part A is the hospital coverage part of Medicare. Most of your parents' hospital bills are covered by Medicare. The Social Security office makes it easy for your parents. They deduct the hospital insurance monthly premium from Mom and Dad's Social Security check and zap it over to the Medicare Trust Fund. Just like any other insurance program, your parents have to kick in for deductibles. As of 2000, they'll pay $776 for a hospital stay of 1 to 60 days. Medicare covers semiprivate rooms, meals, general nursing, and other hospital services. Just about the entire hospital bill is covered by Medicare. Part A will also pay for home health care under certain conditions, durable medical equipment (wheelchairs, hospital beds, oxygen, and walkers), hospice care, and blood transfusions.

2. **Part B.** This is the second part of Medicare known as the medical insurance part. This covers doctors' services, clinical laboratory services, outpatient medical and surgical services, supplies, and outpatient hospital services. Under approved conditions, your parents can also receive home health care services. Mom and Dad pay a deductible of $100 and then *20 percent of the bill.*

Sage Source

To locate your local Social Security office, call 1-800-772-1213 or check out their top-notch Web site at www.ssa.gov.

Hello? Twenty percent of the bill? Yep. Those 20 percents can really add up. It's what everybody refers to as "the gap" (not the store where your kids shop). Just about everybody buys insurance to close the gap and cover the 20 percent that Medicare doesn't. It's known as Medi-gap insurance (more about that in a moment).

Social Security will also automatically deduct Mom's monthly medical insurance premium (Part B) from her Social Security check. She can refuse Part B, but she has to let Social Security know about this. The only reason she should refuse it is if she's under some other plan that covers her medical insurance. She might be getting it from a retiree package, so she doesn't need to pay for the premium. You absolutely do not want to be without this coverage! Many surgeries are being done at outpatient surgi-centers (for example, cataract surgery)—can you imagine paying for this out of pocket?

MEDICARE PART A COVERAGE CHART	
Medicare Part A (Hospital Insurance) Covers:	**What You Pay in 2000* in the Original Medicare Plan**
Hospital Stays: Semiprivate room, meals, general nursing and other hospital services and supplies. This does not include private duty nursing, a television or telephone in your room, or a private room, unless medically necessary. Inpatient mental health care coverage in a psychiatric facility is limited to 190 days in a lifetime.	**For each benefit period you pay:** • A total of $776 for a hospital stay of 1-60 days. • $194 per day for days 61-90 of a hospital stay. • $388 per day for days 91-150 of a hospital stay. (See Lifetime Reserve Days on page 102) • All costs for each day beyond 150 days.
Skilled Nursing Facility (SNF) Care**: Semiprivate room, meals, skilled nursing and rehabilitative services, and other services and supplies (after a 3-day hospital stay).	**For each benefit period you pay:** • Nothing for the first 20 days. • Up to $97 per day for days 21-100. • All costs beyond the 100th day in the benefit period. If you have questions about SNF care and conditions of coverage, call your Fiscal Intermediary.***
Home Health Care**: Part-time skilled nursing care, physical therapy, occupational therapy, speech-language therapy, home health aide services, durable medical equipment (such as wheelchairs, hospital beds, oxygen, and walkers) and supplies, and other services.	**You pay:** • Nothing for home health care services. • 20% of approved amount for durable medical equipment. If you have questions about home health care and conditions of coverage, call your Regional Home Health Intermediary.***
Hospice Care**: Medical and support services from a Medicare-approved hospice, drugs for symptom control and pain relief, short-term respite care, care in a hospice facility, hospital, or nursing home when necessary, and other services not otherwise covered by Medicare. Home care is also covered.	**You pay:** • A copayment of up to $5 for outpatient prescription drugs and 5% of the Medicare payment amount for inpatient respite care (short-term care given to a hospice patient by another care giver, so that the usual care giver can rest). The amount you pay for respite care can change each year. If you have questions about hospice care and conditions of coverage, call your Regional Home Health Intermediary.***
Blood: Given at a hospital or skilled nursing facility during a covered stay.	**You pay:** • For the first 3 pints of blood if you do not replace it.

* New Part A and B amounts will be available by January 1, 2001.

** You must meet certain conditions in order for Medicare to cover these services.

*** Call 1-800-633-4227 to get the telephone number for the Fiscal Intermediary or Regional Home Health Intermediary in your state.

If you have general questions about Medicare Part A, call your Fiscal Intermediary.

Services covered by Medicare, Parts A and B.

239

MEDICARE PART B COVERAGE CHART

Medicare Part B (Medical Insurance) Covers:	What You Pay in 2000* in the Original Medicare Plan
Medical and Other Services: Doctors' services (except for routine physical exams), outpatient medical and surgical services and supplies, diagnostic tests, ambulatory surgery center facility fees for approved procedures, and durable medical equipment (such as wheelchairs, hospital beds, oxygen, and walkers).	**You pay:** • $100 deductible (pay once per calendar year). • 20% of approved amount after the deductible, except in the outpatient setting.
Also covers outpatient physical and occupational therapy including speech-language therapy.	• 20% for all outpatient physical, occupational, and speech therapy services.
Outpatient mental health services.	• 50% for most outpatient mental health. **See note below.**
Clinical Laboratory Service: Blood tests, urinalysis, and more.	**You pay:** • Nothing for Medicare-approved services.
Home Health Care**: Part-time skilled care, home health aide services, durable medical equipment when supplied by a home health agency while getting Medicare covered home health care, and other supplies and services.	**You pay:** • Nothing for services. • 20% of approved amount for durable medical equipment.
Outpatient Hospital Services: Services for the diagnosis or treatment of an illness or injury.	**You pay:** • 20% of the charged amount (after the deductible). During the year 2000, this will change to a set copayment amount.
Blood: Pints of blood needed as an outpatient, or as part of a Part B covered service.	**You pay:** • For the first 3 pints of blood, then 20% of the approved amount for additional pints of blood (after the deductible) if you do not replace it.

* New Part A and B amounts will be available by January 1, 2001.

**You must meet certain conditions in order for Medicare to cover these services.

Note: Actual amounts you must pay are higher if the doctor does not accept assignment (see page 100). If you have general questions about your Medicare Part B coverage, call your Medicare Carrier (see pages 92-93).

Just like Part A, there are certain periods of time when you can enroll in Part B. The general enrollment period is from January 1 through March 31 of every year. Coverage won't start until July.

As you deal with the world of Medicare, there are two different groups you will probably encounter. Here's who they are and what they do:

- **Peer Review Organizations (PRO).** The federal government pays a group of doctors and other health care experts to monitor and improve care given to

Medicare patients. This group will review your parent's complaints about such things as care they've received at a hospital, a hospital's outpatient clinic, nursing home, surgi-center, or home health agency. The PRO will even handle complaints from Medicare managed care plans. Whenever your parents go into the hospital, they'll receive a pamphlet telling them how to make a complaint and the phone number of the PRO to call.

- **Fiscal Intermediary.** Companies are hired by the federal government to pay all Medicare Part A and Part B bills. The feds contract with different companies throughout the country to pay the bills. Sometimes you'll need to call one of these companies to correct a bill or let that company know that something's wrong. The company's phone number appears on the "Explanation of Benefits" or a "Medicare Summary Notice" your parents get after they receive a service from a health care provider that billed Medicare.

Covering the Gap: Medi-Gap

Okay, back to the 20 percent that Medicare doesn't cover for medical services. Dad can buy a Medi-gap insurance policy that will cover the 20 percent. It is vital that he gets this insurance—unless he chooses to get into a Medicare managed care (HMO) plan. As soon as he's receiving his Medicare Part B insurance benefit, he should be applying for a Medi-gap policy.

To make life easier, there are 10 standard Medi-gap plans from which to choose. Get ready for alphabet soup: They range from A (very basic) to J (the whole ball of wax). Of course, the more coverage, the more you pay. Two of the standardized plans that companies can offer to sell your parents can bear the title Medicare SELECT. These policies are less costly; however, your parent can *select* only from the plan's hospitals and doctors.

Sage Source

To search and compare Medi-gap policies and for tips on buying policies, visit www. medicare.gov/MGCompare. Get a free copy of the *Guide to Health Insurance for People with Medicare* at this Web site or call 1-800-633-4227 to order. SHIP (Seniors Health Insurance Program) counselors offer free health insurance advice and can help you sort through Medicare. Call your local area agency on aging (listed in the blue pages of your phone book) to contact your local SHIP program.

The federal government has a first-rate Web site where you can find out what Medi-gap policies are offered in your parents' area (see the following Sage Source). You can identify what kind of coverage you want, and then you'll get a reading of what insurance company offers what you want. You can also get a printout that compares different plans with each other. It's called Medi-gap Compare.

Buying a Medi-Gap Policy

You need to be careful buying Medi-gap policies; here's what you want to watch out for:

- Buy only one plan. It's illegal for insurance companies to sell you a second Medi-gap plan.
- Watch out for clauses that exclude pre-existing conditions. Shop for a plan that will cover your parents' conditions.
- Be careful when you switch plans. Make sure that you're switching for better coverage at an affordable price.
- Make sure the insurance plan can be delivered in 30 days.
- Don't let anyone scare your parents into buying a policy or use high-pressured tactics.
- Request that the insurance company show you verification that it has been approved by the state insurance department to sell its policies. The state approval means the company meets the standards to sell a Medi-gap policy.
- Don't pay cash! Pay by check so that you have proof of purchase. Know who you're dealing with—get a business card.

Senior Alert

When mom and dad hit 65 years old and right after they have enrolled in Medicare Part B, they have six months to buy a Medi-gap policy. During this open enrollment period the insurance company cannot deny your parents coverage or change the price of a policy because of past or current health problems. If your parents don't buy it during that six-month window, insurance companies can deny them a Medi-gap policy and charge them more. So now you know what to buy your parents for their sixty-fifth birthdays!

- If your parents are confused or overwhelmed in making insurance decisions, go over the information with them or have them talk to a SHIP counselor.

- Once your parent decides to buy a policy, fill out the medical history section *very carefully*. If you omit any information, the company will use this as a reason to *not* cover a bill linked to the condition you didn't report.

- Stay clear of nonstandard plans. Insurance companies can't call it a Medi-gap plan if it hasn't met government standards and been approved by your state insurance department.

Out in the Cold: What Medicare Doesn't Cover

Medicare does a great deal, but it doesn't cover everything. Here's what's not covered:

- Almost all outpatient prescription drugs
- Routine physical exams
- Routine eye exams
- Custodial care (help with bathing, dressing, using the toilet, eating)
- Most dental care and dentures
- Routine foot care
- Hearing aids
- Orthopedic shoes
- Cosmetic surgery (got to keep the wrinkles)

You can, of course, shop around for other insurance to pay for some of these services. Medicare *may* cover the first 100 days of nursing home care if it follows a three-day hospital stay and meets other conditions. Then, you're on your own.

What's This About Assignment?

A term you're going to hear plenty about is *assignment*. Medicare assigns how much it will pay for services for a given condition or procedure. If a doctor takes as payment in full the amount that Medicare assigns, then that means the doctor takes "assignment." It also means that your parent doesn't have to pay anything out of pocket. In other words, assignment is a good thing. You want it. Always ask first whether a physician takes assignment.

If the doc doesn't take assignment, your parents will have to pay the difference between what Medicare and the Medi-gap policy cover and what the doctor charges. About three out of every four doctors take assignment. Even if they don't, they can charge only 15 percent more than what Medicare assigns for that service. So, say, for instance, that Medicare assigns $100 for a given service; the doc can charge only $115 dollars. Remember, routine physical exams are not covered by Medicare—so there's no assigned amount. The doc can charge whatever he or she wants.

Senior Alert

If you think your parent has been a victim of fraud or you seriously suspect Medicare is being ripped off (which means we're all being ripped off), call the Office of Inspector General's Hotline at 1-800-HHS-TIPS (1-800-447-8477). Be sure to have on hand the provider's name and any identifying number on the bill, your Medicare number, date and item of service you are questioning, the amount approved and paid by Medicare, and the reason why you suspect a problem. You could qualify for a $1,000 reward!

Original Medicare or Medicare Managed Care?

Now that managed care is on the scene, Mom and Dad have a choice: they can stay in the original Medicare program—the one I've just described to you (sometimes referred to as fee-for-service Medicare) or they can join a managed care organization (HMO). Great. More choices, more decisions.

Sage Source

The Medicare Web site at www.medicare.gov also helps you compare managed care programs. You can also ask for a free copy of their report on quality and customer satisfaction of Medicare managed care plans by calling 1-800-633-4227.

If your parent doesn't mind being treated by an HMO's network of physicians, clinics, and hospitals, then there are some real advantages:

- Your parents can drop their Medi-gap coverage. They do *not* drop Medicare Part A and Part B!
- Preventive care like routine doctor exams, dental care, hearing aids, glasses, and prescription drugs are usually covered.
- The HMO handles all the paperwork.
- At a minimum, they *must* offer everything that the original Medicare offers.

Your parents may also pay a monthly premium to the HMO which is usually less than what they paid for the Medi-gap policy that they dropped.

If your parents see doctors who are already in the plan, don't require a lot of specialists or a particular specialist not in the plan, or live in two different places during the year—this might be ideal and it will save them money.

In Medicare managed care your parents must use the doctors, hospitals, therapists and nursing homes in the HMO's network. They must also receive pre-approval for these services. The HMO decides who, what, where and when. If your parents turn out to be dissatisfied, they can re-enter the original Medicare. They will also need to re-enroll into a Medi-gap policy. Be advised that if Mom or Dad has a new health condition, he or she may have trouble getting back into the old plan or finding coverage for this new pre-existing condition.

Senior Alert

Medicare managed care companies can quit Medicare. They apply every year to Medicare for the right to offer their plan to consumers and can decide not to re-apply. Doctors can join or leave a managed care organization at any time. Even though your mom and dad can re-enter original Medicare at any time, they may have trouble getting their Medi-gap policy back. If it was through no fault of their own—for example, the company they were with quit Medicare—your parents should not be penalized.

How Does Medicare Managed Care Work?

Medicare pays the HMO a set amount of money for the year to take care of your parent. Whatever money they don't spend on your parent, they keep. Of course, like any insurance company, they're hoping that most of their members stay pretty healthy. That way, their outlay is low. On the other hand, if your parent is very ill, they absorb the costs. If your parents are in Medicare managed care, you have to stay on top of it. Some hospitals around the country are dropping out of plans, saying that the managed care companies aren't giving them enough money. In that case, if your parents live in an area where there's only one hospital, they have to shuffle quickly to find an alternative plan.

A New Alternative: Private-Fee-for-Service Plans

And to make things even more complicated, Medicare has just approved a new choice. Private-fee-for-service plans can now be offered by private insurance companies. Medicare will give them a monthly amount, and the private insurance company will provide health care coverage on a pay-per-visit arrangement. The insurance company, rather than the Medicare program, decides how much your parents pay for the services they get. Check out www.medicare.gov to get a free copy of *Your Guide to Private-Fee-for-Service Plans.*

MEDICARE PART B PREVENTIVE SERVICES CHART		
Medicare Part B Covered Preventive Services	**Who is covered...**	**What you pay...**
Bone Mass Measurements: Varies with your health status.	Certain people with Medicare who are at risk for losing bone mass.	20% of the Medicare-approved amount after the yearly Part B deductible.
Colorectal Cancer Screening: · Fecal Occult Blood Test - Once every 12 months. · Flexible Sigmoidoscopy - Once every four years. · Colonoscopy - Once every two years if you are high risk for cancer of the colon. · Barium Enema - Doctor can substitute for sigmoidoscopy or colonoscopy.	All people with Medicare age 50 and older. However, there is no age limit for having a colonoscopy.	No coinsurance and no Part B deductible for the fecal occult blood test. For all other tests, 20% of the Medicare-approved amount after the yearly Part B deductible.
Diabetes Monitoring: Includes coverage for glucose monitors, test strips, lancets, and self-management training.	All people with Medicare who have diabetes (insulin users and non-users).	20% of the Medicare-approved amount after the yearly Part B deductible.
Mammogram Screening: Once every 12 months.	All women with Medicare age 40 and older.	20% of the Medicare-approved amount with no Part B deductible.
Pap Smear and Pelvic Examination: (Includes a clinical breast exam) Once every three years. Once every 12 months if you are high risk for cervical or vaginal cancer, or if you are of childbearing age and have had an abnormal Pap Smear in the preceding three years.	All women with Medicare.	No coinsurance and no Part B deductible for the Pap Smear (clinical laboratory charge). For doctor services and all other exams, 20% of the Medicare-approved amount with no Part B deductible.
Prostate Cancer Screening: • Digital Rectal Examination - Once every 12 months. • Prostate Specific Antigen (PSA) Test - Once every 12 months.	All men with Medicare age 50 and older.	Generally, 20% of the Medicare-approved amount after the yearly Part B deductible. No coinsurance and no Part B deductible for the PSA Test.
Shots (Vaccinations): • Flu Shot - Once every 12 months. • Pneumonia Shot - One may be all you ever need, ask your doctor. • Hepatitis B Shot - If you are at medium to high risk for hepatitis.	All people with Medicare.	No coinsurance and no Part B deductible for flu and pneumonia shots if the doctor accepts assignment (see page 100). For Hepatitis B shots, 20% of the Medicare-approved amount after the Part B deductible.

As of January 2003, Medicare also covers annual glaucoma screening.

An Ounce of Prevention ...

Medicare does cover some very important preventive exams that should be on every parent's calendar. Don't let your parents follow the old adage, "What you don't know won't hurt you." In these instances, what you don't know can kill you. Make sure your parents get these screenings. There's no excuse not to.

Fighting for Your Rights

Your parents have the right to appeal any bills they have received or decisions that have been made regarding their care as related to Medicare. Here are three things you should know:

- If your parents are in the original Medicare program and they think that Medicare should have paid for, or didn't pay enough for, an item or service your mom or dad received, then your parent can appeal it. On the back of the "Explanation of Medicare Benefits or Medicare Summary Notice" are the directions on how to file an appeal.

- If your parents are in a managed care plan, they would have received directions when they enrolled on how to file an appeal. If you think your parents' health could be seriously harmed by the company's decision, ask for a fast response. By law, the company must answer you in 72 hours.

- If you think your parent is being told to leave the hospital too soon, ask the hospital for the number of the Peer Review Organization (PRO). While the PRO reviews your case, the hospital cannot force your mom or dad to leave.

The Other "M": Medicaid

Medicaid is a health insurance program run by states for people living at or below poverty. The state and the federal government both share the costs. Many older people who qualify for Medicaid are also eligible for the federal government's Supplemental Security Insurance program (SSI). If your mom or dad never held a job, received extremely low wages, or didn't work long enough to qualify for Social Security, he or she may be eligible for SSI. In fact, anyone receiving SSI is automatically enrolled into Medicaid.

Who's in Charge?

Your state department of welfare or human services usually administers the program through local board of assistance offices. Since each state has its own set of rules and policies, check with your local welfare office (in the blue pages of your phone book) to see if your parent is eligible. Under Medicaid, your parents will have access to physicians who accept Medicaid and they will not have to pay a premium or deductibles. Hospitalizations, prescriptions, and doctor visits are covered. Be aware, however, that some doctors, because of the low reimbursement rate given by Medicaid, may refuse to see your parents.

Your parents' home, car, personal belongings, household furniture, and any life insurance policies with a cash value of $5,000 or less *cannot* be counted as assets by the welfare office when it determines your parents' eligibility into the program.

If Mom or Dad is a Medicaid beneficiary, she or he should always send medical bills to Medicare first. Whatever Medicare doesn't cover, the state Medicaid program will pick up.

Spending Down

You might hear the term "spending down" in reference to Medicaid. This is related to nursing home care. Your parents might have entered a nursing home as "private pay" using their savings, assets, and income to meet the monthly bill. At some point, Mom or Dad might spend all of his or her assets, and the lowered income subsequently qualifies your parent for Medicaid. For more information on Medicaid and nursing homes, see Chapters 15, "Choosing a Nursing Home," and 16, "Living in a Nursing Home."

Help with Premiums

Even if your parents do not qualify for Medicaid they may qualify for two state programs that can help them pay their Medicare premiums. If your Mom or Dad can't afford paying the Medicare premiums for Parts A and B and the deductibles, they may be eligible for what's known as the Medicare buy-in program (the Qualified Medicare Beneficiary, or QMB, program). With this program, your parents have to be at or below poverty. If they are, the state will cover Medicare premiums, deductibles, and most of their co-payments. Poverty level means that their financial assets (not the house) can't be more than $6,000 for a couple and $4,000 for an individual.

If Mom and Dad are just above the poverty level (up to 10 percent above), the state will pay for their Medicare Part B premium. This program is known as the SLMB program (Specified Low-Income Medicare Beneficiary program).

Call your local area agency on aging to find out how to apply in your state. The www.medicare.gov Web site offers you the latest eligibility criteria for each program.

The PACE Program (Programs of All-Inclusive Care for the Elderly)

PACE is an optional benefit under both Medicare and Medicaid that wraps long-term care services together for older people who are frail enough to meet their State's standards for nursing home care. The program offers comprehensive medical and social services that can be provided at an adult day health center, home, and/or inpatient facilities. For most clients, the all-inclusive service package enables them to continue living at home rather than enter a nursing home. A team of health professionals will assess your parent's needs and develop a care plan. PACE is available only in states that have chosen to offer PACE under Medicaid. To find out if your parent is eligible or to find out if there is a PACE site available for your parent, call Eldercare Locator 1-800-677-1116 or go to www.medicare.gov/Nursing/Alternatives/PACE.asp for PACE locations and telephone numbers. Half the states as of 2003 offer PACE.

The Least You Need to Know

- Medicare is the federal health insurance program that covers most hospital and physician care for people 65 years and older, disabled persons, and people with end-stage renal disease.

- Medi-gap policies pick up the 20 percent difference between what health care providers charge and what Medicare pays. Your parents should not be without this insurance.

- Medicare assigns how much they will pay doctors for their services. Always ask the doctor if he or she takes "assignment," otherwise you have to pay the difference between what the doctor charges and what Medicare pays them.

- Your parents can opt to belong to a Medicare managed care plan, a private-fee-for-service plan, or they can remain in original Medicare.

- If your parents are of low income, they may qualify for Medicaid (the state-administered health insurance program), the federal Supplemental Security Insurance (SSI) program, or two programs that help pay Medicare premiums and deductibles (QMB or SLMB).

- Stay current on changes to Medicare—bookmark and visit their Web site at www.medicare.gov often.

Chapter 22

The *Saving Private Ryan* Generation

In This Chapter

- Veterans must enroll to receive health care
- Long-term care services for your parent
- Insurance and pension benefits
- Burial and memorial benefits
- Help in finding old comrades

Every year when my dad needs to re-enroll for his Medi-gap policy he calls me up. "Are you sure I can't drop this policy? I'm a vet, they'll take care of me." My dad, like many other veterans, thinks that if he needs hospital care or a nursing home that the Veterans Affairs (VA) system will come to the rescue.

It's not that they don't want to. It's just that the numbers are staggering. There are over nine million veterans aged 65 years or older, and in just 10 years, they will account for almost half of the entire veteran population. On any given day, over a half million veterans need some form of long-term care.

The Veterans Affairs Administration offers a wide array of services that can be very helpful to your dad. And since many of our dads (and moms) are veterans of World War II, I thought a chapter on what the VA system offers would prove pretty helpful.

New Rules: Dad's Got to Enroll

You can't just sit back and think that the VA is going to come knocking or that when your dad wants to receive services he just shows up. In 1996, Congress passed the Veterans Health Care Eligibility Reform Act stating that any veteran who wants to receive VA health care services must now enroll. Veterans can enroll by filling out VA Form 10-10EZ. They can get the form by …

- Visiting, calling, or writing a local VA care or benefits office. VA services are listed in the blue pages of the phone book under "U.S. Government."
- Calling the VA Enrollment Center at 1-877-222-VETS.
- Ordering the form online at www.va.gov.

Your dad will need to have a copy of his DD-214 (Honorable Discharge Certificate). Once your dad enrolls, he will be assigned one of two eligibility categories and a priority ranking.

Geri-Fact

Even though I use the term Dad throughout this chapter, let's not forget the women who served in WWII. In their honor you should know that …

- Over 350,000 women served during WWII.

- The Women Airforce Service Pilots (WASPs) weren't recognized for their valor (38 died in the line of duty) until 1977 by the U.S. Congress.

- The Women's Army Corps (WACs) served all over Europe, North Africa, and the Pacific. Nearly 2,000 received medals for meritorious service, 16 received the Purple Heart, and 200 army nurses lost their lives in the war.

The first category is a "must do" group. The VA must provide hospital and outpatient care to veterans who have a service-connected disability, and to former POWs, World War I veterans, and low-income veterans. Depending upon funding, the VA may also offer nursing home care to this group as well. The disability is graded and given priority levels. Low income is determined by an income eligibility test known as a means test.

The second category is a "may do" group. The VA may provide health care services, depending on the resources the VA has, and the veteran agrees to pay a co-payment for the care.

There are seven priority groups that the VA assigns to veterans who have enrolled for VA health care benefits. For example, vets with a service-connected disability that is 50 percent or more disabling, are given a priority group 1 status. Many veterans among the WWII generation fall into the priority group 5 ranking, which means they do not have a disability connected to the war but their annual income and net worth are low income as determined by the VA system. If your dad is not low income and is not disabled, he is near the bottom of the priority list. He is still eligible for services, but he will pay a co-payment.

VA Health Care Benefits Package

The VA now offers a uniform benefits package. This is a standard health benefits plan that is generally available to all enrolled veterans regardless of priority group. This does not mean that it's free if you have a moderate income. The care is provided on an "as needed" basis that is determined by the VA system. Needed care is defined as "care or services that will promote, preserve, and restore health."

Veterans accepted for enrollment in the VA health care system are eligible to receive necessary inpatient and outpatient services, including preventive and primary care. According to Veterans Affairs, these include …

- Diagnostic and treatment services.
- Rehabilitation.
- Mental health care and substance abuse.
- Respite and hospice care.
- Prescriptions as part of VA treatment.
- Emergency care in VA facilities.
- Hospital (medical and surgical) and outpatient care.
- Prosthetics and orthotics.

Prescriptions are covered when veterans receive their treatment from a VA medical facility. Most of the time, the veteran will be asked to pay a $2 co-payment. Generally, hearing aids and eyeglasses are not covered when the hearing and vision loss is due to aging.

Geri-Fact

Veterans of World War II dominate the landscape of our parents' generation. Consider these facts:

- Of the 16,535,000 soldiers who fought in World War II, six million are alive today.
- There are over 3,000 living veterans from World War I.
- Nearly three million Presidential Memorial Certificates have been given to surviving family members in honor of their loved ones' military service since JFK began the tradition in 1962.
- The National Cemetery Administration maintains more than 2.3 million gravesites throughout the United States and Puerto Rico.

Long-Term Care Services

The VA system does offer a wide range of services to meet your dad's long-term care needs through 1,000 locations of care throughout the country. Here's a brief description of what the VA provides *directly:*

VA Long-Term Care Services	Description
Nursing home	VA nursing homes are hospital-based, providing nursing, medical, rehab, psychosocial, and pharmaceutical care; the VA runs 131 nursing homes.
Home-based primary care	The VA provides primary care in the home to severely disabled, chronically ill vets; the VA provides medicines, equipment, supplies, and home improvements to accommodate living at home.
Adult day health care	This is a therapeutic outpatient day program for frail, elderly vets, providing health maintenance and rehab; there are fewer than 20 such programs.
Respite care	Caregiving relatives can place a chronically ill and disabled vet in a VA hospital or nursing home for a brief period of time.
Domiciliary care	This is a residential rehab and health maintenance center for veterans who don't require hospital or nursing home care but are unable to live alone because of physical or psychiatric disabilities.

If They Don't Have It, They'll Get It

The VA system will contract out their long-term care services to other agencies, *if* they are not able to directly deliver the service to your dad. So, if your dad needs nursing home care, home health care, adult day health care, or domiciliary care, or your mom needs respite care and the VA can't provide it directly, it will pay for the services provided by another organization to your dad or mom. For example, in 1997 the VA contracted with 3,700 nursing homes in the community to care for over 6,000 veterans. So, just because there isn't a VA medical center in your community doesn't mean that the VA can't help your parents. Of course, your parents will need to meet the VA's eligibility criteria.

Senior Alert

The hospital-based nursing homes of the VA system are very expensive to operate. So is paying for over 7,000 veterans' nursing home stays in the community. The law allows the VA to pay for community nursing home care for up to six months for conditions that are *not* connected to military service. However, the six months are not a given. In fact, many report that only 30 days of care are provided. The major purpose of nursing home care is to provide a transition from the hospital to the community. The length of stay, however, may be longer for those with service-connected conditions. Bottom line: Don't expect the VA to pick up Dad's nursing home care indefinitely.

State Veterans Homes

These "old soldiers' and sailors' homes" as they are known in many communities, are actually a partnership between the VA and the states. The state operates the homes; however, the federal VA system approves them, pays for up to 65 percent of the construction costs to build them, and subsidizes a portion of the daily cost of care. There are nearly 90 state-run veterans' nursing homes in 39 states. You must go through your state to gain admission into these homes. Most state homes require eligible veterans to share the cost of their care. It's best to call the home directly to find out its eligibility rules.

Alzheimer's/Dementia Program

The VA system offers three types of inpatient dementia units: The first provides a comprehensive diagnostic unit; the second is a behavioral unit that offers up to

90 days of treatment for behavioral as well as physical problems; and the third is a long-term care unit that provides comfort and care for vets in their final stages of the disease. Outpatient clinics are also provided by the VA for diagnostic workups and treatment. About one third of VA health care facilities offer dementia programs.

Geriatric Research, Education, and Clinical Centers (GRECCs)

These centers integrate research, education, and clinical practices in geriatrics and gerontology. What researchers and medical practitioners learn at these centers they impart to the whole VA system. As of 1999, there were 20 such centers nationwide, with federal funding to suport five more. If your parent is fortunate enough to live near one, it can provide Dad with excellent, comprehensive care. To find out a GRECC located near you, visit their Web site at slcgrecc.med.utah.edu/greccweb, or go to the senior health services section of the VA Web site at www.va.gov.

Silver Lining

Your dad may be eligible to purchase VA life insurance. These policies are for a maximum face amount of $10,000. Under certain conditions the premium may be waived due to total disability. Veterans whose policies participate in dividends can increase their coverage beyond the limit by using the dividends to buy additional coverage. Call 1-800-669-8477 to speak to a VA insurance specialist or visit www.insurance.va.gov.

Cancer Care

The Department of Veterans Affairs and the National Cancer Institute have developed a partnership that offers veterans wide access to clinical trials (research studies) on cancer. These trials take place at VA medical centers and outpatient clinics throughout the country. You can call the Cancer Information Service at 1-800-4-CANCER or visit the VA Web site at www.va.gov/cancer.htm to find out if and where a clinical trial is available for your dad. Of course, cancer trials are available outside of the VA system, as well. Clinical trials offer free medical services for patients who have a condition that researchers want to study. Usually they are testing the benefits, side effects, and problems with certain drugs or medical practices. The benefit is that your parent receives free care; the downside is that it is experimental and there can be negative side effects.

Burial and Memorial Benefits

It's been a long-standing tradition of the United States military to honor its dead. Arlington National Cemetery, the Tomb of the Unknown Soldier, the Vietnam Memorial, and the Memorial Day holiday are all hallmarks of this honor. There are a number of burial tributes and benefits that can be comforting to you, your mom or dad, and your family.

Burial at a Military Cemetery

The VA has a National Cemetery Administration that maintains 118 national cemeteries in 39 states. The VA determines eligibility to be buried at a national cemetery. To determine eligibility, call 1-800-827-1000. There are also state-run veterans' cemeteries. These have similar eligibility criteria as the national cemeteries, but usually require residency in the state. You can get contact information for your state and an overview of the steps you need to take for burial in a national cemetery by going to the VA Web site (www.va.gov). Upon request, you can also receive a military head marker.

Sage Source

The procedures to get burial benefits and copies of the forms are available at the VA Web site (www.va.gov); just click on Burial and Memorial Benefits. You can also call 1-800-827-1000 or write to the U.S. Department of Veterans Affairs, National Cemetery Administration (403A), 810 Vermont Avenue, NW, Washington, DC 20420. Your funeral director is probably also aware of the benefits and can help make arrangements for you.

Burial Expenses

The VA usually pays a funeral allowance of $300 for funeral expenses and may also pay transportation costs for the remains. A claim must be filed within two years of the death. When death occurs at a VA facility, nursing home, or nursing home under contract with the VA, the burial expense benefit is usually available.

Military Funeral Honors

The Department of Defense, as of January 1, 2000, is responsible for an "Honoring Those Who Served" program that provides military funeral honors to veterans. Families must request this service; your funeral director should ask you if you want it and make the contact for you. A military funeral ceremony consists of two or more uniformed military persons coming to the gravesite to play "Taps" and present the family with the United States burial flag. While I was writing this book, my stepfather, a World War II veteran who received the Purple Heart, died. I can't tell you how much it meant to my mother and his children to have a military funeral for him. It was a solemn and cherished moment for all of us when my mother was presented with the U.S. flag to honor the service of Samuel J. Baressi.

Presidential Memorials and Burial Flags

A Presidential Memorial Certificate (PMC) is an engraved paper signed by the President to honor the memory of honorably discharged veterans who have died. The certificate recognizes your dad's "devoted and selfless consecration to the service of our country." More than one certificate may be provided so that each next of kin can receive a copy. To receive one, you can apply in person at a VA regional office or send a request by mail. You will need to include a copy of the veteran's discharge documents and your return address. There is no form to fill out. (See the previous Sage Source sidebar for the address.)

The VA gives out nearly a half-million burial flags every year to honor deceased veterans. You can obtain one from the VA regional offices and most U.S. post offices. You'll need to fill out VA Form 2008 and submit a copy of the veteran's discharge papers. You can download the form from the VA Web site (www.va.gov).

If your dad has lost his discharge papers, click on Requests for Veterans' Military Information at the VA Web site.

Silver Lining

Your dad or mom probably has quite a story to tell about his or her service during World War II. These are important stories to pass on. Check out the following Web sites on creating an oral history:

- **www.muscanet.com:** This Web site focuses on the role of women during the war. There's a terrific oral history on "What Did You Do in the War, Grandma?"

- **www.tankbooks.com:** This Web site has wonderful stories, great links, and interview examples on how to ask your veteran parent about the war to create an oral history for your family.

Tracking Down Old Buddies

Okay, enough with this depressing death stuff. Lately, your dad might have been talking about how great it would be to hook up with his old military unit. My dad, who was stationed in Italy, talked about it for years and by chance found a reunion announcement in *The Legion* magazine. He went to his reunion. It became a mile marker in his life and a reason to tell his children and grandchildren stories about the war. If you'd like to help your dad find his comrades, go to the VA Web site's Burial and Memorial Benefits section and click on Locating Veterans. And if you need a reason to get motivated, rent the movie *Saving Private Ryan* or read Tom Brokaw's book, *The Greatest Generation* (Random House, 1998).

The Least You Need to Know

- Your dad must enroll to receive any health care benefits from the VA health care system.

- The VA can provide home health care, primary care, nursing home care, and dementia care at VA centers.

- If the VA can't provide the service directly, it can contract for the service with other agencies. Your dad doesn't have to live near a VA medical center to receive long-term care services.

- Most honorably discharged veterans can receive a wide range of burial and memorial benefits.

- The VA has an excellent Web site to help your mom or dad track down old comrades. Visit it at www.va.gov.

Chapter 23

Beating Out-of-Pocket Expenses

In This Chapter

- Saving seniors money on doctors' visits, prescriptions, and more
- The skinny on long-term care insurance
- How to find a good insurance company
- What to look for in a policy
- What about travel insurance?

No more kids to raise, no more college tuition, and often, no more mortgage ... sounds like you should be rolling in the green stuff! But most older folks will tell you that despite their new-found financial freedom, a new set of expenses quickly fill the void. And they run up against a ceiling—no more unlimited earning potential without a job.

Life in the retirement lane is a fixed one. Your parents' new set of expenses are the medical ones that are rising far faster than Mom and Dad's Social Security and retirement checks. Last year the cost of prescription drugs increased by 17.4 percent despite the fact that the annual inflation rate was under 2 percent. Deductibles, home health care, and prescriptions have a heyday with your parents' annual income. Add home repairs coupled with high utility bills, and that mortgage-free home looks downright expensive.

But there are many things you and your parents can do to beat the out-of-pocket expenses that attack the geriatric wallet. In this chapter I'll show you some options you may not have considered.

Smart Consumer Tips

Ever buy one of those travel books, *Europe on Ten Dollars a Day* or *100 Free Things to Do in New York?* It's pretty amazing what's out there when you know where and how to look for it. In the following sections we take a closer look at several ways you can cut down expenses.

Doctors Who Take Assignment

One of the first questions you should ask your parent's physician is whether or not he or she accepts Medicare assignment (see Chapter 21, "Got to Have Those M&Ms: Medicare and Medicaid," for a refresher course). If the doctor does, it means he or she will accept the amount paid by Medicare as payment in full, even if the doctor's bill is normally higher. If your parent also carries a Medi-gap policy, they won't have a balance to pay the physician. Just about three out of four doctors take Medicare assignment. Of course, your parent still must pay his or her annual Medicare deductible.

Senior Alert

Routine doctor office visits and physicals are not covered by Medicare. A physician can charge whatever he or she deems necessary. Ask up front how much the doctor charges for routine services.

If the doctor doesn't accept Medicare assignment, he or she is permitted to charge your parent up to 15 percent more than what Medicare would have paid the doctor. So, if Medicare would have paid the doctor $100, he or she can charge no more than $115.

Whether the doctor accepts assignment or not, you must pay 20 percent of the bill. Medicare pays 80 percent of the assigned amount for a procedure. That's why most people carry a Medi-gap policy to take care of the 20-percent "gap."

Free Shots

Flu shots can literally be a lifesaver for your parents, especially if they have any pulmonary problems. Rather than pay $35 for an office visit and another $15 for the shot, your parents can get the shot for free. Most seniors' centers offer flu shots prior to flu season and so do many local public health centers. A good number of hospitals also offer flu shots as a community service. Your local area agency on aging should know who is offering flu shots; give them a call at 1-800-677-1116.

Senior Discounts

Businesses large and small want a share of the older market, thus the explosion of discounts offered to those who are 55-plus. You'll find plenty of grocery stores offering senior-discount days as well as free delivery to regular customers. Internet buying through groups like Priceline.com can allow you to shop for Mom and Dad from your home and get them discounts. Pharmacies usually offer at least a 10-percent discount to seniors who pay cash for their prescriptions. Even utility companies offer discounts to older customers; some offer reduced rates for those who are at a moderate to low income. During heat waves when air conditioners are in high demand or during severe cold spells, many utility companies allow seniors to pay their bills over longer periods of time.

Besides discounts, your parent can get free screenings for a number of health conditions (although these screenings should not be substituted for routine physicals). Many of these are offered at malls; ask for the mall's calendar of events at the information desk usually located in the center of the mall, or call the mall's main number. Local hospitals and senior centers also offer free screenings on a regular basis. Just about every line of business offers some sort of senior discount, just ask.

Secondhand Equipment

Many senior centers have programs in which previously used wheelchairs, quad canes, walkers, crutches, and other durable medical equipment can be leased for a small donation. If your senior center doesn't have such a program, call the local area agency on aging (1-800-677-1116) to track down an organization that may offer this service. You can also check out your Yellow Pages under Secondhand Stores. Remember, if the equipment is prescribed by your physician, Medicare will cover the costs, so be sure to check with your physician.

Generic Drugs

I discussed prescriptions at length in Chapter 8, "Pills and Your Parents," but it's worth reminding you here that your parents can save on prescriptions if they buy the generic version of a brand drug prescribed by their physician. Generics can cost half as much as brand drugs,

Geri-Fact

According to a recent study by Rutgers University's Division on Aging, elderly Americans spend 19 percent of their total income on out-of-pocket medical expenses annually. That's one out of every five dollars. Half of these dollars are spent on drugs and dental care. People who report poor health spend much more on out-of-pocket medical expenses, as much as one third of their income.

and they must be approved by the FDA as being therapeutically equivalent. So ask your doctor about getting a generic and tell the pharmacist you want it. For more on saving money on prescriptions, see Chapter 8.

Volunteer Services

Throughout this book you've been directed to all kinds of community services that are available to you. Before you pay for things like companion services, cab rides, respite care, catered meals, chore services, and minor home repairs, call your local church or synagogue or area agency on aging to see whether they provide such services or know of any organization that will for a small fee or donation. These services, of course, are for those with a modest income.

Long-Term Care Insurance

Long-term care insurance is something that both baby boomers and their parents should consider. If your parents are 80-plus, it's really too late to be of any value. If they're in their 60s and early 70s, listen up.

Long-term care insurance is rather new to the insurance scene. We're all used to life insurance, car insurance, and disability insurance (you might not realize it, but if you're working, Uncle Sam has you covered through Social Security). The whole deal with insurance is to protect yourself against a major loss that you can ill afford. Bottom line: You don't want to take the risk. Insurance companies know that lots of people are just like you. So they ask large numbers of people to pay a set amount of money (the more the better) and they'll take the risk for you. They, of course, hope you're a lucky soul and they'll never have to pay out. The more the risk is shared, the less everybody needs to chip in.

Geri-Fact

If your parents are 65 years and older, they have a 43 percent chance of requiring nursing home care at some point in their lives. Half of all elderly women will probably use nursing home care before they die. One out of five of those who enter nursing homes will be there for five years; half are there for one year.

How Much Does It Cost?

The problem right now with long-term care insurance is that the numbers of people buying into it are still pretty small. In fact, less than 1 percent of all the money spent on long-term care in this country is paid from a long-term care policy! So, without a large base to spread the risk, the premiums are pretty high. Prices range from $3,000 to $8,000 per year, depending on the kinds of benefits you pick, how long a waiting period you choose before the benefits kick in, and how many years of nursing home coverage you choose.

Enter the chicken-and-the-egg game: Not until more people join up will the insurance premiums come down. Not until the premiums are lower will more people join up. In the meantime, the costs of long-term care can bankrupt many American families. The average nursing home costs $50,000 per year. Can you handle $1,000 a week?

Why Buy Long-Term Care Insurance?

When you think of it, the odds of needing nursing home care are a lot higher than losing your house to fire, totaling your car, or being so disabled you can never work again. Yet, we don't think of being without car insurance or homeowners insurance. Why the hang-up over long-term care insurance? Well that's not too hard to figure: Who likes to think about old age or nursing homes? Who likes buying insurance? Besides, when people do think about it, they're convinced that Medicare covers nursing homes or the state will pick up the tab. Wrong on the first count, and you better be poor on the second count. On top of all this, you're feeling sandwiched: Everyone's on your case to put money aside for your kid's college bills and sock money away for your retirement. And you're to do this while you're paying a mortgage, car loans, and just plain having a life. So what should *you* do? And what should your parents be doing when it comes to long-term care insurance?

There are five major reasons why people buy long-term care insurance:

- To maintain their independence so they won't have to rely on family members
- To protect their assets against the high costs of long-term care; to preserve their children's inheritance
- To make long-term care services affordable, such as home health care and custodial care
- To provide themselves with more options than just nursing home care, and to pay for nursing home care if it's needed
- To preserve their standard of living

If any of these reasons strike a chord with you and you know that one year of nursing home care or intensive home health care (about two-thirds of the cost of nursing home care) would slam your family's resources, you should seriously consider getting a policy. This is especially true if your parent does not want to deplete his or her estate by paying for care and/or there is a strong history of debilitating illnesses in the family (stroke, Parkinson's, Alzheimer's) that often point to long-term care.

Finding a Good Insurance Company

When researching an insurance company to provide long-term care insurance (or any kind of insurance), the first thing you want to do is make sure the company is financially solid, with an excellent reputation in its service delivery. There are four rating companies that issue grades on insurance companies; A.M. Best is well known, as is

Standard and Poor's. Don't take a policy with company that has lower than an A rating. Because long-term care insurance is still a relatively new product, and because insurance companies are still guessing at how much it will really cost them to cover long-term care, choose an insurance company that can absorb paying out more claims than it had forecasted. Rating directories of insurance companies are available online.

Sage Source

One Web site that's a must-visit is www.insure.com. *U.S. News & World Report* and *Money* magazine voted this site as a best on insurance and as a "Best of the Web" site. It has excellent material on insurance, including a Complaint Finder that reports an insurance company's record by state. You'll find specific news on your state and a link to your state's department of insurance. It also taps Standard and Poor's insurance rating data bank. For A.M. Best's ratings online, visit its Web site at www.ambest.com.

What You Should Look for in a Policy

As with buying any insurance policy, it's buyer beware (and be aware). You need to study these policies well and know exactly what you are buying. Long-term care isn't simply nursing home care. It's care your parent will need for the long haul as opposed to a short three-day stay in a hospital. As you've learned throughout this book, there are a wide range of options your parent can choose from all under the heading of long-term care. So what should you look for?

What Kind of Care Is Covered?

Long-term care policies usually offer one or all of the following kinds of long-term care:

- **Nursing home care.** This is a public or private facility that provides intermediate and skilled nursing care. Some nursing homes also provide custodial care and assisted living. They are licensed by the state and are monitored by the federal government if they accept Medicare. Not all facilities are Medicare certified.

- **In-home care.** This is care provided in your own home. There's a range of products that the insurance company can offer you in this area. Ask which of these are part of the company's basic policy and which are add-ons that you'll have to pay more for on your premium. Typical services are skilled nursing care, home health aides, and homemaker assistance.

- **Respite care.** This provides temporary care for the insured person to give a family member, who is providing in-home care on a daily basis, a break from his or her caregiving responsibilities.

- **Hospice care.** This provides care for those who are terminally ill. (Note: Medicare provides hospice care coverage, so make sure you're not overinsuring yourself or your parents on this benefit.)

Most companies have created three levels of care that they apply to their long-term care products: skilled care requires doctors, nurses, and registered therapists; intermediate care requires trained personnel who are under the supervision of a doctor or nurse; and custodial care requires nonmedical personnel to help with the tasks of adult daily living.

Of course you will want the nursing home coverage. The question will be for how long (we'll get to this in a few minutes). The real question at this point is to decide what other long-term care services you want. Most policies now cover home health care as part of their basic package. You usually have to pay extra for custodial care, homemaker service, and respite care. So, take a good look at the policy and make sure it specifies which services are extra and which are basic.

If your mom is recovering from a bad case of the flu, she might not need a registered nurse, but she could definitely use someone to come in to cook, get her prescriptions filled, give her a bath, monitor her health, and alert someone if Mom needs to get to the doctor. This would come under custodial care. I highly recommend making this part of your package. It's the "stitch in time saves nine" factor.

Whatever you do, make sure the agent clearly spells out what the company defines for each level of care and who decides if that level of care is needed. Most companies require that your parent cannot perform at least two adult daily living (ADL) tasks before the coverage kicks in (eating, bathing, using the toilet, walking, dressing). Companies frequently send out a company nurse to assess your parent's condition. Ask the agent about any restrictions surrounding hiring help (whether you can hire a relative, for instance). Does your parent have to be assessed first? What is the appeal process if you disagree with the level of care decision the company made?

What's a Reasonable Reimbursement Rate?

Call several nursing homes in your area and find out what their daily rate is. Then call a few home health agencies and find out what they charge per hour for home health care (not custodial care). Average the rates out; that will give you a ballpark figure for knowing the maximum amount you want your insurance company to cover you for. Say, for instance, the average rate in your area for a day in the nursing home is $120 and you think your dad could afford $30 a day for two years, then he'd want a policy for $90 per day. The higher the rate, the higher your premium.

Inflation Protection

Here's something you've got to watch out for and demand. If you need nursing home care 10 years from now and the rate you've settled on is $100 per day, it might cover you up to lunch in another decade! So, if you're in your 50s or 60s, you'll want a policy that allows for at least 5 percent annual inflation compounded annually. Now, if your mom is getting this policy in her early 70s, inflation protection isn't as important because, in all likelihood, she will use it a lot sooner.

Silver Lining

Pick a policy that will allow your parent to redirect his or her benefits between the home care and nursing home care amount. For example, if your dad exhausts all of his nursing home care benefit but he never tapped the amount reserved for home health care—and it's clear he'll never use it— the company would redirect the home health pot into his nursing home bill.

Coverage for Alzheimer's and Dementia

Here's where you can get into a word game with the insurance crowd. When long-term care insurance was first introduced, many companies didn't cover people with Alzheimer's. Hello? Nearly half of all nursing home residents have Alzheimer's or another form of dementia. Most companies reconsidered and now cover it. But not everybody who has dementia or cognitive impairment has Alzheimer's. It's too restrictive a definition. *You're better off with a company that includes "cognitive impairment" in its policy and accepts a broader definition of dementia.* Cognitive impairment involves problems with someone's attention, memory, or other thinking functions so much so that the person cannot be left alone. The condition can be reversible, so you don't want a policy that limits coverage to cognitive impairment that is only irreversible.

The Waiting Game

The fewer days you have to wait to receive benefits, the higher the premium. Since Medicare will *usually* pay for the first 100 days of nursing home care, you can hedge your bets with the insurance company and opt for a 100-day waiting period before it kicks in with nursing home care. But remember, you'll still need a Medi-gap policy to cover the 20 percent that Medicare won't pay for. You are also taking a gamble: There are certain requirements that must be met before Medicare pays for nursing home care; it's not guaranteed (see Chapter 21).

Now, waiting for 100 days before you can get home health care coverage is a whole other story. You've either gotten a lot better or a lot worse after 100 days. Look for different waiting periods for the home health care portion of your coverage.

Are There Eligibility Requirements?

Find out if the insurance company requires your parent to be hospitalized prior to receiving home health care benefits or nursing home care, if a company nurse performs an assessment before your parent receives care, and if any doctor can prescribe the care. The hospitalization requirement can trip you up—not everybody goes from a hospital to a nursing home.

What's the Maximum, and for How Long?

Policies are usually sold offering one-, two-, three-, five-year, and lifetime benefits, getting progressively more expensive as the years pile on. You'll have to decide on the maximum number of years you can afford based on the premium. Once you've exhausted the number of years you chose, it's over. Some companies offer a lifetime maximum; other policies pay for nursing home care per episode with a designated break between each benefit period. Some companies might pay for 150 days, require a 60-day break, and then start up again. Be very clear on what you're deciding.

Waivers and Guaranteed Renewals

A waiver of a premium will allow your parent to stop paying his or her premium payments once Mom or Dad has begun to receive benefits. Again, companies will vary on how soon this provision will takes effect. Some insurance companies allow it to take effect immediately; others might require you to continue paying premiums for 180 days. You also want to make sure that the company gives your parent

Silver Lining

Some states have a partnership going between the insurance industry and Medicaid. People who buy long-term care insurance that covers them for a set period of time can go on Medicaid without losing their assets. Contact your state insurance department to see if your state has such a program. You can find the directory of all state insurance offices by visiting www.insure. com.

Geri-Fact

According to 1995 statistics, the average overall length of stay for those who enter nursing homes at 65 years is approximately 888 days. The breakdown of older age groups looks like this: The length of stay for those 65 to 74 is 1,064; for those 75 to 84, 864 days; and for those 85 and over, 713 days.

"guaranteed renewability," which means the only reason it can cancel your parent's policy is because Mom or Dad stopped paying the premium. If your parent isn't good about paying bills, have the company send you copies of the bills so you can stay on top of it and make sure the bill is paid.

Fixed Premiums for Fixed Incomes

If Mom or Dad can afford a policy that provides a fixed premium, it will be much better for your parent if he or she is on a fixed income. Insurance companies can raise rates; however, it has to be across the board for all the policy holders. An insurance company cannot target your parents just because they submit a claim, as it can do when your teenage son has his second traffic violation.

Upgrade Privileges and Nonforfeiture Protection

It's smart to find a policy that allows you to upgrade its benefits. The long-term care industry is in a constant state of evolution and there might be a service five years from now that you'll want. When it comes to nonforfeiture, you're looking for a policy that gives you back some of the value of the policy should you decide to cancel it. Be aware that this provision will definitely increase the price of your premium.

Pre-Existing Conditions and Exclusions

This is everybody's favorite bone to pick with the insurance industry. Be up front about any conditions that your parents have when you apply for the policy. It does not pay to lie! You want a policy that will cover the pre-existing conditions because it's likely that those conditions will result in need for long-term care. Some companies will specify a period of time (for example, six months or a year) before they'll cover a certain condition. Make the insurance company spell out all exclusions in simple terms.

Sage Source

The Shopper's Guide to Long Term Care Insurance, developed by the National Association of Insurance Commissioners (NAIC), includes a worksheet to help you compare policies. To order this guide, write to NAIC Publications, 2301 McGee Street, Suite 600, Kansas City, MO 64108 (phone: 816-783-8300; e-mail: pubdist@naic.org). Ask for it by title or by publication number: LTC-LP.

A Word on Travel Insurance

If your parent is doing quite well and plans to jaunt around Europe or any place outside the United States, tell Mom or Dad to take out travel insurance. Medicare stops at the U.S. boundaries! So, if Mom gets any medical care in another country, she'll have to pick up the tab. (Talk about a lovely souvenir!) Some policies will also cover any down payments made for a trip that Mom had to cancel due to an illness.

These pearls of wisdom come from my mother-in-law, who recently became ill during a cruise. She was rerouted from the cruise ship to a clinic in Greece for five days. Fortunately, she had insurance. The insurance company even flew her back to the States with a doctor.

The rate for travel insurance is usually based on the cost of the trip, coming in at around a few hundred dollars. Given the out-of-pocket expenses you could incur being sick abroad, this is a pretty smart investment.

The Least You Need to Know

- There are lots of ways your parents can save on out-of-pocket expenses, such as using generic drugs, looking out for senior discounts, and taking advantage of free flu shots and health screenings.

- Long-term care insurance can protect your parent's life savings, but do your homework before you buy a policy!

- If you purchase long-term care insurance, make sure it covers home health care services and care rendered if your parent should have Alzheimer's disease.

- If your parent travels outside the United States, he or she should consider investing in travel insurance. Medicare is not applicable outside the United States.

Planning for Incapacity

None of us likes to think about death. Or losing control. Or having Alzheimer's disease. Or ending up in a coma. Nor is it high on our list to talk any of this over with our parents. We don't want to appear as if we're trying to take control over their lives or their finances. Yet, the truth of the matter is, dealing with potential incapacity while our parents are *well* keeps them in control rather than takes it away.

Death isn't very simple these days. Medical technology and drugs have teamed up quite well in saving and prolonging our lives. It is not uncommon for people to recover from strokes and heart attacks. Cancer is rarely an immediate death sentence—chemotherapy can buy years. And pneumonia, which used to be considered the "dying old man's best friend," can easily be banished. But too much of a good thing can also mean your dad lies in a vegetative state, hooked up to machines that breathe for him. Or it may mean a paramedic arrives at the house to perform CPR on your mom, who is dying from late-stage Alzheimer's.

Candid and compassionate discussions about what your mom and dad want when they're no longer able to make decisions for themselves will preserve their dignity and control and keep peace in the family. Now who wouldn't want all that?

What's an Advance Directive?

Advance directives are legal documents that spell out your parents' wishes regarding future medical care and treatment. It is based on two major principles of law: A person has the right to accept or refuse treatment (informed consent), and a person has the right to appoint someone to act on his or her behalf. Advance directives are in effect immediately and—most importantly—when the maker of the advance directive (your parent) is no longer able to make decisions for him- or herself.

Advance directive is actually a general term. There are two types of advance directives: a living will and durable health care power of attorney. Let's take a closer look at each one.

Living Will

A *living will* is a type of advance directive in which your mom states her wishes as to whether or not she wants medical treatment that will prolong her life should she become terminally ill or injured, or permanently unconscious. The living will takes effect when a doctor determines that death is fairly certain or that the person is in a persistent vegetative state with virtually no hope of recovery. The document tells the doctors, hospital, and other health care providers exactly what your mom wants to have done or not.

Every state has its own law regulating living wills. Most states have adopted specific living will forms for you to use. States also identify under what conditions the living will is considered valid. Since state laws can change at any time, it's important that you use a current form and become aware of your own state's laws surrounding this kind of advance directive.

If your parent (or you) is interested in writing a living will, here are two excellent resources:

- **Aging with Dignity,** a nonprofit organization dedicated to promoting better care of the dying and human dignity, offers a terrific Five Wishes advance directive that serves as both a living will and durable health care power of attorney. You can view a copy on that organizations Web site (www.agingwithdignity. org) and have it mailed to you. This form has been accepted by 33 states, which are identified on the form. It's very easy to understand. Contact Aging with Dignity, P.O. Box 1661, Tallahassee, Florida 32302; 1-800-562-1931.

- **Choice in Dying, Inc.,** a nonprofit organization, fosters communication about complex end-of-life decisions. They provide advance directives, counsel patients and families, train professionals, and act as advocates for improved laws. At their excellent Web site (www.choices.org) you can download each state's living will forms, keep current on end-of-life issues, and track down related resources. Contact Choice in Dying, Inc., 1035 30th Street, NW, Washington, D.C. 20007; 1-800-989-9455.

Most living wills have statements that release doctors from any legal liability for withholding medical treatment that would prolong the patient's life. As you can imagine, doctors and hospitals fear lawsuits from family members who charge they haven't done everything possible to save a life. If your parent doesn't have a living will, doctors will go full swing into, a life-saving mode, as you see in the TV show *ER*.

Your parent must face one central question: "How much medical intervention do I want to keep me alive when death is certain?" There are a number of responses to that question. On the following page are some of the medical treatment issues you and your parent should discuss when completing a living will.

Sage Source

If you want to write your own living will, pick up a copy of *How to Write Your Own Living Will,* by Edward A. Haman (see Appendix A, "Resources," for more information). All the forms for every state are included with easy-to-understand directions. Good background information is also provided in this excellent book.

Senior Alert

A living will is worthless if it's secretly stored away in a safety deposit box. Here's who should get copies: your parents' primary family physician and specialists, you and other family members, the person who is their agent (an individual chosen by your parents to make health care decisions on their behalf should they become incompetent), the hospital that they would be taken to in an emergency, and any nursing home they are admitted to. If they are very active in their church or synagogue, share a copy with the priest, minister, or rabbi. Always take a copy of the form whenever your parent is being treated at a health care facility (such as an outpatient surgery center).

Medical Treatment Decisions for a Living Will

When his or her condition is terminal and death is certain, does your parent want …

1. Cardiac resuscitation (CPR)?

_____

2. Mechanical respiration (breathing machine)?

_____

3. To receive food and water via a feeding tube or intravenously when he or she can no longer eat or swallow?

_____

4. Blood products (transfusions)?

_____

5. Any surgery or invasive diagnostic tests?

_____

6. Kidney dialysis?

_____

7. Antibiotics?

_____

8. To be taken to the hospital?

_____

9. Life-sustaining treatment stopped if it has been started?

_____

It is also important to spell out in the living will what your parent does expect from medical caregivers. For example: Mom doesn't want to be in pain; she doesn't want anything done to intentionally end her life; she wants to be kept clean and warm and offered food and water by mouth.

Not all living wills specify the need for a surrogate decision maker on your parent's behalf. If a living will is very thorough with specific instructions, a surrogate won't be necessary.

Your parents will need to sign their living wills in front of witnesses. Each state specifies who are considered acceptable witnesses, so be sure to find out your state's rules.

It's a general rule of thumb that witnesses should not be family members, health care providers, or anyone with a financial stake in your parents' estate. Some states require the living will to be notarized. Even if they don't, it doesn't hurt to have the will notarized anyway.

Durable Health Care Power of Attorney

So what's the difference between a durable health care power of attorney and a living will? The living will centers on end-of-life decisions. The medical treatments called into question focus on sustaining life when there's no hope for recovery or death is certain.

The *durable health care power of attorney* is broader than a living will. It empowers the agent to make health care decisions on behalf of your parent *any time* your parent becomes incompetent. The agent can make decisions on admissions and discharges to and from health care facilities, what to do with medical records and organ donations, whether or not to move the patient, make arrangements for home health care and accept or refuse treatment that affects the physical and mental health of the patient. Furthermore, these medical decisions are for all levels of health care—not just focused on impending death.

Geri-Fact

DNR orders stand for "do not resuscitate." This notation is written by a physician on a patient's medical record. It lets all health care staff know that if the patient stops breathing or his or her heart stops beating, no one will try to revive the patient. The DNR term might also be referred to as a "no code" order. DNR orders can also be given to EMTs (also known as emergency medical technicians or paramedics) to release them from the obligation to resuscitate. You must show them, however, an executed legal document. You can call Choice in Dying at 1-800-989-9455 to get a copy. By law, a person must be resuscitated unless the health care staff are given the executed legal document specifying otherwise.

Again, each state has its own laws governing durable health care power of attorney. Many documents granting this right also have a living will section.

Here are some of the basic tenants of durable health care power of attorney:

- You don't have to be a lawyer (whew!) to be designated as having durable health care power of attorney on behalf of your parent. The word "attorney" simply means "designated agent."

- The power of attorney does *not* kick in until your parent is legally *incompetent!* As long as Mom and Dad are competent, they make the decisions.

- Your parents must be competent when they complete and execute the durable health care power of attorney papers. This will not be considered legal if you're doing this at Dad's bedside after he's just suffered a major stroke or has been diagnosed with Alzheimer's. If there's any question regarding your parent's competency, see a lawyer. You may need to get a written opinion from a doctor.

- When a patient is unable to give informed consent (such as during anesthesia), the durable health care power of attorney takes effect.

- Many states have laws that spell out procedures for determining when someone is legally incompetent. You and your parent should be familiar with what is required. Usually physicians and lawyers become involved in this determination.

You might find that your state refers to the durable health care power of attorney by different names, such as health care proxy, health care agent, medical power of attorney, or attorney-in-fact. For more information and forms regarding durable health care power of attorney, contact Aging with Dignity or Choice in Dying, Inc. (see the "Living Will" section earlier in this chapter for contact information).

Silver Lining

If your parents change their minds and want life-sustaining procedures done, living wills and a durable health care power of attorney can be revoked. For most states, people can execute a new living will that cancels out their old one, or state in writing that they revoke their current living will. Copies of this statement should be given to anyone who received the former living will. To avoid any debate, get the new will notarized.

Federal Law: The Patient Self-Determination Act

In 1991 Congress passed the Patient Self-Determination Act, requiring that patients be told of their right to accept or reject medical treatment in advance while they are competent. Any agency receiving federal money is required to inform you and your parent of this right. Since just about everybody—hospitals, nursing homes, home health agencies—gets federal money, they all have to inform you of this right. They also are required to give you information on their policies with regard to advance directives and living wills and the state's laws governing these policies.

When your parent is admitted to a hospital, Mom or Dad will be asked whether he or she has a living will or durable health care power of attorney. If so, the hospital staff will place the documents in your parent's patient file.

In case of an emergency, always bring the advance directive (living will and/or durable health care power of attorney) with you. If your parent lives alone, you can always send the papers to the hospital to have them on file in case of an emergency.

During an emergency, things will get very hectic. Don't hang back and assume that someone is in charge of finding out whether or not your parent has a living will—let them know immediately!

General Power of Attorney

Your parents may decide that they want to give you or someone else more general powers to make decisions on their behalf. Perhaps they are away six months of the year and want you to pay bills and make decisions regarding the property. They might want to authorize you to sell the house, invest their savings, or conduct all their financial affairs.

Other than clearly spelling out what powers have been granted, this type of power of attorney should also stipulate whether or not it's in effect should your parents become legally incompetent. If this isn't specified, your powers are no longer valid when your parents become incompetent. This type of legal document should involve a lawyer to help your parents clearly state their wishes and their expectations. Whoever is designated as your parents' agent should also clearly understand what is expected of the agent and should require protections from liability as long as the agent acts in good faith.

Senior Alert

Make sure all family members know and understand your parents' intentions with their advance directives. Everyone should get a copy. If a hospital knows of just one family member disagreeing with the others and is pushing for life-sustaining treatment, the hospital will probably err on the side of caution and initiate treatment to avoid a lawsuit.

Guardianship—Are You Sure?

If your parent severely lacks the capacity to make any decisions on his or her behalf, or has become a real danger to him- or herself and others, you face a tough set of issues. Perhaps Mom has suffered a severe stroke and there is no chance for recovery, or Dad's been diagnosed with Alzheimer's disease that is progressing rapidly. In these instances, your parent is no longer competent to grant you the powers of attorney previously discussed.

Seeking guardianship, however, is something you do as a last resort. It is a public court proceeding that imposes demanding rules and tests to determine your parent's capacity to make decisions. You will need to retain a lawyer who will petition the court. The court will appoint a lawyer to represent your parent. Interviews will be conducted with those involved with your parent's care (for example, the family physician); you might bring expert testimony such as the results of a geriatric assessment, or the court may order such an assessment. Your parent will be informed of the hearing and can attend if he or she wants to.

Every state has its own laws governing guardianship. These laws can be rather complicated and might change, thus the need for a lawyer. You'll also find that most states have different levels of guardianship. Limited guardianship, for example, provides the guardian authority over certain limited conditions. For example, Dad may not be capable of handling any of his finances but is capable of making decisions about who takes care of him at home. In most states, guardians usually report to the court at specified times to update the court on how things are progressing.

If your dad is declared incompetent or incapacitated by the court, he is stripped of his right to vote, sell property, execute finances, determine his living arrangements and medical treatments, drive, or enter into any type of contracts. Hopefully, you won't have to go down this path, but if you do, work with a lawyer. Informal agreements among family members can turn sour very quickly, leaving you open to a wealth of legal problems and even accusations of elder abuse.

Just What Is Death, Anyway?

At the very core of all these decisions is how death is defined. In your parent's younger days, that used to be a pretty simple venture. Death was determined when the heart simply stopped beating. After the heart ceased to function, it didn't take long for all other organs to follow suit and shut down. But today, breathing machines and CPR have literally brought people back from the dead. With the invention of respirators, the lungs are given air mechanically, blood continues to flow, the heart keeps pumping, and the brain gets its oxygen. So, technically, even if the heart can't beat on its own, it still beats. Thus, under the old rules, you're not dead. Now what? The experts had to scramble to find a new way of defining death. They came up with *brain death*. Surprise! The center of our life is not our hearts but our brains (not a good development for Cupid).

Geri-Fact

Brain death is the irreversible loss of brain function needed to sustain basic life processes such as respiration and circulation.

Two kinds of brain death can occur: the first is cerebral death, which means that the upper portion of the brain no longer functions, leaving the person in a coma often referred to as a persistent vegetative state. In this instance, the brain still sends signals to keep breathing and circulation going but hardly anything else. In the second kind of brain death, the lower part of the brain commonly known as the brain stem ceases to function. In this instance, the most primitive and elemental functions of the brain cease—the signals to breathe, circulate, and control temperature. The person must be kept on a respirator to maintain life.

No matter how death is defined, the final reality leaves broken hearts (and sometimes, relief that a loved one's suffering is over). Your mom and dad can help ease some of the pain by taking it upon themselves to make the tough life and death decisions *now* rather than have their children wrestle with them.

The Least You Need to Know

- The best way that your parents can control their lives when they are incapacitated is through an advance directive. Advanced directives are not an age thing; everyone should have them.

- A living will spells out your parents' wishes as to what life-sustaining measures they want and do not want should they become terminal and incapacitated. A durable health care power of attorney allows an individual appointed by your parents to make health care decisions on their behalf should they become incapacitated.

- The Patient Self-Determination Act requires that patients be told of their right to accept or reject medical treatment in advance, while they are still competent.

- A general power of attorney is used if your parent wants to give you general powers to make decisions on their behalf. It's best to have a lawyer spell out the areas of decision-making your parent is granting.

- Guardianship is used as a last resort to take nearly all decision-making away from your parent due to proven lack of capacity.

- Brain death is the irreversible loss of brain function needed to sustain basic life processes such as respiration and circulation.

Chapter 25

Lawyers, Wills, and Estate Planning

In This Chapter

- Elder law attorneys
- Talking to your parents about estate planning
- Wills and letters of instruction
- The three types of trusts
- The probate process
- The role of an executor/executrix

Despite "the best-laid plans," things can go wrong in life. But without laying down *any* plans, the likelihood of more going wrong than right is pretty darn high.

This chapter is about your parents laying down plans to protect their assets, pass on an inheritance, and plan for their care if they become incapacitated. It's about them remaining in control, and when life throws them a bad curve, how to get the legal resources to fight it.

The New Legal Beagles: Elder Law Attorneys

Over the last 10 years there's been a crop of new lawyers bursting onto the legal scene: elder law attorneys. As the ranks of older people have grown, so has a new field of services and products targeted to the geriatric set. Demands have been high for these services while resources have been limited: enter the world of appeals.

Elder law attorneys help thousands of older people appeal denials of Medicare, Medicaid, Social Security, and a wide range of insurance claims. They can also assist in estate planning, probate, and administration and management of trusts. Or you might want them to fight for your dad's retirement and pension benefits and make sure your mom receives the survivor benefits due her. These are the guys who can help you with living wills, durable power of attorney, conservatorships, and guardianships. If you suspect abuse of your parent or if Mom or Dad's been scammed, an elder law attorney is the most prepared to take on the bad guys.

Most elder law attorneys have a specialty such as estate planning, or they know the ins and outs of appealing government and insurance denials. Rarely does a lawyer do everything in elder law. The one thing most elder law lawyers bring to their practice is the knowledge and sensitivity of working with older clients. They have gained an appreciation and insight as to the needs of the elderly and how the "system" can work for them or against them. Health care laws in Medicare, Medicaid, and health care insurance are complex and frequently change. It's best to get an expert who is up on the latest changes and is savvy to the appeal process.

Finding an Elder Law Attorney

Once you know your problem would benefit from legal expertise, then start calling around to identify someone with a proven track record. Call local associations such as the Alzheimer's Association, the

Senior Alert

Before you hire a lawyer, make sure your parent's problem is a legal one. There may be other organizations that can help if it's a medical or social service issue. Call your local area agency on aging (1-800-677-1116) to see if it (or another organization it recommends) can solve your problem first.

Sage Source

The National Association of Elder Law Attorneys offers a registry of elder law attorneys nationwide. Visit its site at www.naela.com, and you can search for lawyers by specialty and location. You'll get the contact information you need and great links to other legal resources. You can also contact the association at 1604 North Country Club Road, Tucson, AZ 85716; 520-325-7925.

local AARP chapter, geriatric care managers, hospital social workers, or the local senior center. Perhaps your financial advisor or family accountant knows of someone. Your state and local bar association can offer lists of lawyers in your community and their areas of expertise.

What to Ask

Finding the best lawyer for the job means learning to ask good questions. To help you narrow your search, call each lawyer and ask each one (or the lawyer's representative) ...

- How long has the attorney been practicing in general, and how long has he or she specialized in elder law?
- What is the attorney's specialty in elder law?
- What percentage of his or her practice is dedicated to elder law?
- What professional associations does the attorney belong to?
- Is there a charge for the consultation?

Briefly describe your problem, and ask if this is the kind of thing this lawyer works on. Once you've identified the lawyer who best meets your needs, set up the consultation. Be sure to take the time to organize your parent's case prior to the meeting. At the consultation, ask ...

- How do you propose solving my parent's problem?
- Are there any other courses of action? Could you please describe the pros and cons of each?
- How much time do you expect it will take to resolve this matter?
- How much do you expect this to cost?
- Can you project a success rate on such cases?
- Will you be handling this case or will someone else? What is your or the other attorney's experience in this type of case?

Beyond finding a lawyer with solid knowledge and experience, you and your parents want someone that you feel you can trust. Someone who respects your parents and has their interest at heart. Following your consultation, trust your instincts, and keep looking if you feel the lawyer fails in the "trust" department.

Sage Source

For a terrific, up-to-date review of laws, regulations, and legislation that affect seniors, along with a list of resources, check out www.seniorlaw.com.

Talking to Your Parents About Their Assets

From the time we were little kids, my grandmother used to tell me and my siblings that if we didn't behave, we'd be "out of the will" (her version of "time out"). We had no clue as to what a will was, but we figured we wanted to be in it. As we got older, we understood she was just joking, but we also learned that it was taboo to ask her what was in the will. Like most American families, we knew our grandparents and parents wanted to pass things down through the family. We also knew not to talk about it.

Turns out we were in the norm. Many surveys report that the majority of Americans rarely discuss estate planning with their parents. Adult children have no idea of what their parents would want them to do with their wealth if Mom or Dad became incapacitated.

There are three basic reasons why people write wills or create trusts:

- They want to pass their assets on to their family members rather than let government take over their assets.
- They want to keep peace in the family by identifying who gets what before they die.
- They want to plan ahead for the costs of incapacity, including the care of their spouse.

These are all very noble and smart reasons for your parents to write a will, create a trust, and engage in smart estate planning. But what is your role in all of this? If your parents have saved and invested wisely, you really don't have much of a role. If they have not, and you're concerned that they haven't protected their assets, you may need to broach the subject with them.

Here are some suggestions on approaching your parents about their estate planning (or lack of it):

- Begin the conversation with wanting to understand what your parents want; something like, "Dad, I really want to carry out your wishes, but I need to better understand them. Do you want to pass down property to the family? Do you want to be able to draw down money from your assets to help care for you and Mom? Have you thought about ways to avoid high taxes and lengthy probate?"
- Acknowledge that you fully understand that this is *their* money. Advance planning on their part means that they can keep control. Your goal is to help them keep control—not relinquish it to government or strangers in some courtroom.
- Stay focused on your parents' concerns. This is about them—not your needs or wants. Perhaps they're worried that they'll outlive their resources, or that the

kids will fight over the estate and the family will break apart. They may be struggling with finding a fair way of dividing up what they'll leave behind. Rather than confront these issues, they'd rather not talk about them or just plain avoid them altogether.

- If you feel they're uncomfortable talking with you, ask them to see a financial planner.

- One way of approaching the issue more subtly is to share with them your experience of setting up a will or doing your own estate planning: "Mom, you'll never believe what I learned the other day, if I set up a trust I can ...." Or, "I just filled out my living will, and did you know that ..." or "Dad, I want you to know that I named Jeff [husband] as my durable health care power of attorney. This is how it works ..." These create an opening to discuss how your parents have addressed or not addressed these issues.

- Share with them an actual story of how someone who didn't have a will caused his or her children to lose a great deal of their parent's hard-earned wealth through taxes and probate.

- If you know of a smart and better way for your parents to leave you money (for example, via a trust) you might try, "Dad, I don't know what you're leaving me, and that's okay, but you might want to consider setting up a trust so that the money will be protected in case someone should sue me in my work."

Senior Alert

Don't go behind your sibling's back to assist your parents in their estate planning. Your influence—though well meaning—may be interpreted as greed by your brother or sister. If you value your relationship with your sibling, be above board. Fairness is more important to siblings than equally dividing up pieces of the estate. But fairness will be achieved only through open lines of communication.

Money has long been at the root of many a divorce. Fights over how money is spent hits many a household. Tread carefully in bringing this up with your parents. This is *their* money. Your motive ought to be about helping them (if they need the help) meet their needs and wishes regarding the preservation and handing down of their assets. And remember, an inheritance, if you receive one, is a *gift*, not a right.

Where There's a Will, There's a Way

We all know the routine: "I, Janie M. Smith, being of sound mind, hereby bequeath …" and away you go, giving away everything you own. A will is simply a legal document that provides instructions on how your parents want their property to be passed on to their heirs after your parents die. Witnesses (who don't benefit from the will) are needed, and the will must be in writing and clearly dated. Don't consider a will to be written in stone. Families and circumstances change, and so should wills. Many experts recommend that each parent have his or her own will to avoid the complications of a joint one. This holds especially true if your parents have remarried.

Wills usually describe assets, property, and personal possessions and how they are to be distributed after someone dies according to the owner's wishes. Most often the will passes down assets to a surviving spouse and then to children. In a will, your parent needs to identify who will administer his or her estate—meaning pay taxes and outstanding bills, and assure that the instructions in the will are carried out. The person who does this is known as the executor (if a man) or executrix (if a woman). (I'll tell you more about being an executor/executrix later in the chapter.)

Senior Alert

If your parent dies without a will, it's known as dying "intestate." The state then determines the rightful heirs and how much they receive. The state—and Uncle Sam—take a greater chunk of your parent's estate than if he or she had a will. Even probate costs are higher. The courts appoint someone to manage the distribution of your parent's estate—again, for a fee. The bottom line: Everyone should have a will!

Sage Source

Nolo's legal Web site (www.nolo.com) offers you all kinds of resources and access to highly rated books. Suze Orman's Protection Portfolio offers forms for wills, durable health care power of attorney, and revocable living trusts. Go to www.suzeorman.com or order through QVC at 1-800-345-1212. Visit the site or call 1-800-992-6656 to order *Nolo's Willmaker*, a CD that takes you through an easy interview format to complete a will. AARP's Legal Hotline Technical Assistance Project runs 21 senior legal hotlines throughout the country. Call 202-434-2164 or visit www.aarp.org/foundation/hotline.

Letter of Instruction

Often, people will include a "Letter of Instruction" (also known as a "Tangible Personal Property Memo") along with their will. This is an informal, nonbinding letter that describes your parent's wishes that are not included in the will. A letter of instruction is an extra ounce of prevention against family disputes over the "small stuff." Here are some examples of what might be mentioned:

- Who receives pieces of furniture, jewelry, mementos, collectibles (records, baseball cards, books), family china, clothing, plants.

- Arrangements to care for a pet(s).

- Funeral and burial instructions. Who should receive memorial contributions.

- The location of all important legal documents.

- A list of all insurance policies, stocks, beneficiaries, bank accounts, identification of passwords, and PIN numbers.

- Instructions regarding credit cards, mortgages, titles of cars, properties, the location of income tax returns, and a list of debts.

- Instructions regarding business files, software, equipment, and the password to the computer.

- Personal wishes on how your parent would like to see the heirs spend or invest their inheritance.

Sage Source

Two excellent books about wills and inheritance are *The Inheritor's Handbook* by Dan Rottenberg and *The Complete Idiot's Guide to Wills and Estates* by Steve Maple (see Appendix A, "Resources," for information on both).

In Trusts We Trust

Lots of folks think that trusts are for the rich and famous. But that really isn't so. There are basically three types of trusts: testamentary, revocable, and irrevocable living trusts. Let's take a closer look at each.

Testamentary Trusts

A testamentary trust is usually established to hold assets for a specific reason, such as a child's college education. This kind of trust comes into effect *after* your parent's death as spelled out in the will. Your parent's assets are transferred to the trustee as if that trustee were the beneficiary. The trustee's job is to hold the property for the actual beneficiary. Two major reasons people set up this type of trust is to escape taxes and to provide a means to hold assets until a beneficiary reaches the age of maturity.

Revocable Living Trusts

Revocable living trusts are set up during your parent's lifetime. Your parent retains full control of the trust unless he or she becomes incapacitated. A secondary trustee is also designated, often a bank or other financial institution. Should your parent become incapacitated, the secondary trustee will take over and follow the directives your parent has outlined in the trust. This way your parent maintains control. One major advantage is that any property placed in the trust does *not* go through probate (see the section, "What's Up with Probate?" coming up). It also means that if your dad comes down with Alzheimer's, no one has to go through the rigorous legal steps involved in acquiring guardianship. The trust is completely private, whereas wills are public documents. No one can contest a trust as they can a will. Probate costs are avoided. The trust can be revoked by the maker at any time.

Geri-Fact

Here are a few legal terms you should know:

- **Codicil:** An amendment to a will. (Keep copies!)

- **Decedent:** The person who has died.

- **Fiduciary:** Someone who acts on behalf of others.

- **Attorney-in-fact:** Someone who has the legal power to act on behalf of another person. You don't have to be a lawyer.

Irrevocable Living Trusts

Now enter the rich and famous. Irrevocable living trusts are used by people with extremely large estates. And as the name implies, these trusts can't be changed or destroyed. The grantor sets the terms of the trust during his or her lifetime, however, the grantor can't change those terms once they are set in motion. This is as close to setting something in stone as you can get. If your parent is in the position of being able to consider this option, he or she will certainly have the resources to hire lawyers to execute the trust.

What's Up with Probate?

When your parent dies, you need to take Mom or Dad's will to your local county government office that handles *probate*. Some counties call these offices, probate court, registrar of wills, or surrogate's office. Be sure to bring an official copy of the death certificate and your personal identification when you arrive with the will. The court will look over your papers and confirm that they are valid and you, indeed, are the executor. If there is no will, the judge will appoint an executor. All of the stakeholders of the will—creditors, heirs, and beneficiaries—will be given notice that probate has begun. Next step is an inventory and appraisal of the estate. Everyone is paid who is due money—creditors and taxes get first dibs. An accounting of the estate's remains is completed and then the heirs receive their inheritance.

Some people avoid going through the probate process by having "joint tenancy." In this case, you jointly own property with your parent. By law, you as the survivor, own the property upon the co-owner's death. But you'll also be exposed to any judgments against the property and so may your spouse. It's best to talk with a good estate planner to determine whether or not this is best for you and your parent. Life insurance and pension benefits go directly to beneficiaries and/or survivors without going through the probate process.

Geri-Fact

Probate is a court where all the creditors of the person who has died are paid and where the estate is divided among the heirs after death. This is the court that also administers any estates without wills.

On Being an Executor: Honor or Headache?

Some adult children think that the sibling chosen to be the executor is actually given an honor. But before you feel snubbed if you're not picked, here are just some of the things an executor does:

- Inventories all of the assets
- Identifies and lists all of the debt
- Arranges to have all assets and debts appraised
- Notifies creditors that they need to file their claims for payment and pays all creditors
- Files claims with insurance companies
- Opens a checking account from which to pay bills and deposit assets

- Closes old bank accounts
- Pays taxes to the state and federal government and files a final income tax return
- Decides whether or not assets must be sold to satisfy debts
- Distributes the assets as directed in the will

Still think it's an honor? As you can guess, depending on how large or complicated your parent's estate is, this process can literally take years. Compensation is given to the executor out of the estate and in many states the amount is set by law. If you live out of town or have an extremely busy life, it might make more sense to hire someone to act on your behalf. Whether you hire someone or do the work of the executor yourself, you can gain peace of mind in knowing that you've helped your parent close the final chapter in his or her life.

And this brings us to *my* closing chapter. On behalf of your parents, thank you for reading this book. I hope it's taken you on a journey that's given you the tools, insight, and sensitivity to care for them as they age. Giving back to your parents in ways that improve the quality of their lives is nothing less than a gift—to them and to you.

The Least You Need to Know

- Elder law attorneys specialize in legal areas that affect seniors. Their expertise can save your parents time and money.
- Talking with your parents now about their estate planning will save you time and headaches after their death.
- No one should be without a will, and most people should look into the advantages of setting up a trust.
- You can avoid probate costs by establishing a trust.
- Be fully aware of the responsibilities of being an executor.

Resources

Health and Medicine

Alcoholics Anonymous (AA)
Phone: 212-870-3400
Web site: www.alcoholics-anonymous.org

Check your phone book first for a local chapter. AA offers support to alcoholics and their families. Click on "Is there an Alcoholic in your Life?" to help answer questions about family members and loved ones.

Alzheimer's Association
Phone: 1-800-272-3900
Web site: www.alz.org

This is an excellent organization with a Web site that offers you a wide range of information and support services. It provides a caregiver's guide, "ask the expert" online, medical information, and a finder to locate your local Alzheimer's chapter.

Alzheimer's Disease Education and Referral Center
Phone: 1-800-438-4380
Web site: www.alzheimers.org

This site provides the latest information on new treatments; you can track current clinical trials and how to connect to 20 national Alzheimer's disease centers throughout the country. The site also keeps you posted on results of the most recent research studies.

American Diabetes Association
Phone: 1-800-342-2383
Web site: www.diabetes.org

The association's Web site is very extensive, giving you the latest in research, general info, nutrition, news, lifestyle tips, and links to other great sources. On this site you can also find local chapters near you.

American Heart Association

Phone: 1-800-242-8721

Web site: www.americanheart.org

This group provides research, information, and education about the heart. Click on a great site map to see what's available. Includes warning signs of heart attacks and stroke, separate sections on women, patient information, and links to other sites.

The American Lung Association

Phone: 1-800-586-4872

E-mail: info@lungusa.org

Web site: www.lungusa.org

Contact a local chapter by typing in your zip code on the Web site. Search the site for information on all lung topics—asbestos, air quality, tobacco, tuberculosis, etc. View and download free pamphlets.

Arthritis Foundation

Phone: 1-800-283-7800

Web site: www.arthritis.org

This foundation offers very good consumer health information on prevention and treatment of arthritis. It provides information and referral services and can refer you to a local chapter, support groups, and classes by phone or at the Web site. The Web site also has a product store and a section on advocacy.

Healthfinder

Web site: www.healthfinder.gov

This is a gateway site to consumer health and human services information from the U.S. Department of Health and Human Services. It's a great site, easy to use, has links to agencies and databases, and has a directory of services.

The Lighthouse National Center for Vision and Aging

Phone: 1-800-334-5497

Web site: www.lighthouse.org

This center provides very helpful information for those with vision problems and a terrific catalog of devices to make life easier and vision better. It will also tell you where a low vision clinic is near you.

MEDLINEplus

Web site: www.nlm.nih.gov/medlineplus

This is the site for the National Library of Medicine and National Institutes of Health; if you want to bookmark just one site for your medical information, this is it. It's a terrific resource for all kinds of medical information linking you to other resources. Click on the drug information site—you can review reports on over 9,000 prescription and over-the-counter drugs.

National Association for Continence

(formerly Help for Incontinent People)
Phone: 1-800-252-3337
Web site: www.nafc.org

Provides education, information, advocacy, and support for the public and health professionals on incontinence. The Web site includes "10 Warning Signs of Incontinence," a guide to products, and a continence referral service.

National Coalition for Cancer Survivorship

Phone: 877-622-7937
E-mail: info@cansearch.org
Web site: www.cansearch.org

This is a patient-led organization for patients with cancer and their families. The Web site includes a "Help for Caregivers" section with a "Cancer Survival Toolbox" series—listen to audiotapes or view transcripts. Click on *CanSearch: Online Guide to Cancer Resources* for an excellent primer on how to get cancer information on the Web.

National Council on Alcohol and Drug Dependence

Phone: 212-206-6770; 1-800-622-2255 for affiliate referral
Web site: www.ncadd.org

This is a nationwide, voluntary organization dealing with alcoholism and other drug addictions. It provides education and information, along with advocacy efforts. Click on "Publications" to get a copy of the brochure "What are the Signs of Alcoholism?" a self-test to determine if you or a family member needs to discover more about alcoholism.

National Eye Institute

Phone: 301-496-5248
Web site: www.nei.nih.gov

This institute specializes in vision—research and information for professionals, the public, media, and educators. The Web site has everything—a search function, eye charts, online publications, and a great site map.

National Health Information Center

Phone: 1-800-336-4797
E-mail: nhicinfo@health.org
Web site: www.nhic-nt.health.org

This is a multipurpose Web site designed to help the general public and professionals find health information. It includes a listing of health-related organizations, with links, and a year 2000 list of toll-free numbers for assistance.

National Heart, Lung and Blood Institute

Phone: 301-251-1222

Web site: www.nhlbi.nih.gov

Receive excellent information on diseases of the heart, lung, and blood. Learn about the latest results of studies, news, and centers that are seeking patients for clinical trials.

National Institute of Diabetes, Digestive and Kidney Diseases

Web site: www.niddk.nih.gov

The institute offers a wealth of information on these diseases, giving you the latest research results, a clinical trial finder, understandable health information, and links to other helpful sites to prevent and control these diseases.

National Institute of Mental Health

Phone: 301-443-4513

E-mail: nimhinfo@nih.gov

Web site: www.nimh.nih.gov

Get the latest information on symptoms, diagnosis, and treatment of mental illness. Call for brochures, fact sheets, and other materials. On the Web site, click on "For the Public" for quizzes to help see if someone has an anxiety disorder or depression, or to find out more about medications and mental disorders.

National Institute of Neurological Disorders and Stroke

Phone: 1-800-352-9424

Web site: www.ninds.nih.gov

The institute offers a top-notch Web site describing brain attacks and offers prevention strategies. It also offers information on other brain disorders such as Parkinson's, Alzheimer's, and epilepsy. You can also receive referrals to local clinical research centers.

National Institute on Aging

Phone: 301-496-1752

Web site: www.nih.gov/nia/

This Web site includes a resource directory with links to other aging-related sites, as well as a list of "Age Pages" on various topics related to aging available to the public. You can read the "Age Pages" online.

National Institutes of Health

Web site: www.nih.gov

This federal agency houses a wide range of health institutes cited in this appendix. By visiting this gateway site you can link onto other institutes, find clinical trials for most diseases throughout the country, and review the data on 9,000 prescription and over-the-counter drugs.

National Mental Health Association
Phone: 1-800-969-6642
E-mail: infoctr@nmha.org
Web site: www.nmha.org

This is an organization with 340 local affiliates dedicated to improving mental health and conquering mental illnesses. The Web site has an information center to find affiliates and obtain free publications. Click on "Confidential depression-screening test" to gauge your (or a loved one's) sense of depression.

National Osteoporosis Foundation
Phone: 202-223-2226
Web site: www.nof.org

This is a membership organization with a lot of information on the Web site. Get advocacy, news, information for patients, prevention tips, brochures, videos, awareness kits for free and for sale. Since there is no osteoporosis specialty among doctors, the "Find a Doctor" button provides a strategy for finding a doctor.

National Sleep Foundation
Phone: 202-347-3471
Web site: www.sleepfoundation.org

Great information on sleep disorders and treatment. Print out the foundation's "Sleep Journal" so that your parents can keep track of their sleeping patterns and give it to their doctor. You can also find sleep clinics on the Web site.

National Stroke Association
Phone: 1-800-787-6537
Web site: www.stroke.org

The association offers a wide range of information on strokes. It makes referrals to medical experts, rehab centers, and support groups. The Web site offers very good links to other related sites.

Paralyzed Veterans of America
Phone: 1-800-424-8200
E-mail: info@pva.org
Web site: www.pva.org

This veteran's service organization focuses on special needs of veterans with spinal cord dysfunction. Issues include: health care, research, education, benefits, civil rights, and opportunities for paralyzed veterans.

Parkinson's Resource Organization
Phone: 877-775-4111
Web site: www.parkinsonsresource.org

A 10-year-old national organization devoted to helping people affected by Parkinson's disease, it provides information, education, support, and a newsletter.

Self Help for Hard of Hearing People
Phone: 301-657-2248
Web site: www.shhh.org

This nonprofit, educational organization offers very good links and information on hearing loss and hearing aides. It identifies free screening sites throughout the country during annual Hearing Loss Week.

Death and Dying

Aging with Dignity
Phone: 850-681-2010
E-mail: fivewishes@aol.com
Web site: www.agingwithdignity.org

This is a privately funded nonprofit organization that puts a special emphasis on i mproving care for the elderly at the end of their lives. "Five Wishes" is an easy-to-understand living will, or advanced directive, for all ages. Click on "Five Wishes" on the Web site for a preview.

American Hospice Foundation
Phone: 202-223-0204
Web site: www.americanhospice.org

This organization provides you with helpful information on hospice care. Referrals to a hospice near your parent, counseling resources, and support programs are available on its Web site.

Growth House, Inc.
Phone: 415-255-9045
Web site: www.growthhouse.org

This group is billed as the "Internet's leading online community for end-of-life care." It is an award-winning gateway site to resources for life-threatening illnesses and end-of-life care. You get great information and group support through chat rooms.

National Hospice Organization
Phone: 1-800-658-8898
Web site: www.nho.org

News, public policy information, general hospice information, and links to other good sites are offered on this Web site.

Government Agencies and Services

Access America for Seniors
Web site: www.seniors.gov

This is: "… a government-wide initiative to deliver electronic services from government agencies and organizations to seniors." A one-stop Web site for anyone who wants information on senior issues—from A to Z. Link to your state's aging site.

Administration on Aging
Web site: www.aoa.gov

This is the federal agency that acts as the hub for all government aging services and provides the network of state and area agencies on aging. The Web site is chock full of information and links to other related government sites.

Department of Veterans Affairs
Phone: 1-800-827-1000
Web site: www.va.gov

This federal agency operates all of veteran's services. The Web site is excellent and will save you a great deal of time. You can determine your parents' benefits, who qualifies for what, and how to apply. Contact information is provided and application forms can be downloaded and printed.

Eldercare Locator
Phone: 1-800-677-1116
Web site: www.aoa.dhhs.gov/elderpage/locator.html

This service is run by the National Association of Area Agencies on Aging. If you call and describe your problem, someone will direct you to local and regional agencies for senior services and to your local area agency on aging. You can also receive this info by visiting the Web site.

Housing and Urban Development (HUD)
Phone: 888-569-4287
Web site: www.HUD.gov/senior.html

This federal agency runs low-income housing for seniors. Visit its Web site to find out if your parent qualifies for federal congregate housing and other housing services.

Medicare Hotline
Phone: 1-800-MEDICAR (1-800-633-4227)
Web site: www.hcfa.gov or www.medicare.gov

Call the Medicare Hotline to inquire about plans and what HMOs offer service in your area, to get brochures mailed to you, or to complain about problems or report fraud. At www.medicare.gov you can click on "Nursing Home Compare" and get the latest inspection reports on every nursing home in the country.

Social Security Administration (SSA)
Phone: 1-800-772-1213
Web site: www.ssa.gov

SSA is the federal agency that runs Social Security retirement, survivor's benefits, disability insurance, and SSI (Supplemental Security Income). The Web site is an award-winning government site, easy to use, and answers most of your questions. It offers a directory of local offices.

Caregiving Resources

Please find aditional caregiving website info in Appendix E.

Children of Aging Parents
Phone: 1-800-227-7294

This is a national nonprofit group offering information and referrals. It is listed in almost every guide or resource directory that lists caregiving referral and information resources. Call for information on all caregiving questions.

National Association of Professional Geriatric Care Managers
Phone: 521-881-8808
E-mail: info@caremanager.org
Web site: www.caremanager.org

An association of member geriatric professionals, with an emphasis on advocacy, education, and standards of care for the elderly. Click on "Care Management Resources" for a very good list of Web site links, with a description of each Web site accompanying the link to help you in your search.

National Family Caregivers Association
Phone: 1-800-896-3650
E-mail: info@nfcacares.org
Web site: www.nfcacares.org

This is a national charitable organization for caregivers. It provides assistance in the areas of information and education, support and validation, and public awareness and advocacy. Its Web site is comprehensive.

National Federation of Interfaith Volunteer Caregivers
Phone: 1-800-350-7438
Web site: www.NFIV.org

This is a nationwide alliance of 1,300 faith-based, community-based programs. Volunteers help people remain independent, and provide respite for families who are caregivers. Call the toll-free number to get connected with a local chapter or visit the Web site.

General Resources

AAA Foundation for Traffic Safety
Phone: 1-800-305-7233
Web site: www.aaafts.org

A foundation focused on driver education, safety, and prevention. Order free brochures on driving and the older driver or buy videotapes about older drivers and safety issues. Several written driving tests for the older driver can help families deal with difficult issues.

Abledata—Assistive Technology
Phone: 1-800-227-0216
Web site: www.abledata.com

This is an organization that provides catalogs of information about assistive technology. Product information price ranges are included on the Web site. The National Institute on Disability and Rehabilitation Research of the Department of Education funds the site, but it does not endorse any of the products.

American Association of Homes and Services for the Aging
Phone: 202-783-2242
Web site: www.aahsa.org

Represents 5,000 not-for-profit facilities that care for the aging and those in assisted living. The Web site has a section designated "For Consumers and Family Caregivers." Search by city, state, zip, and type of facility or service to find a not-for-profit nursing home, assisted living facility, or community-based service.

American Association of Retired Persons (AARP)
Phone: 1-800-424-3410
Web site: www.aarp.org

An educational and action organization for those 50 and older. The Web site is excellent. To find caring for an aging parent info, type the word "caregiver" into the search box. AARP members can take advantage of the AARP Legal Services Network (www.aarp.org/lsn), a free first consultation with a lawyer.

Center for Medicare Advocacy
Phone: 860-456-7790; 1-800-262-4414 in Connecticut; 202-216-0028 in Washington, D.C.
Web site: www.medicareadvocacy.org

This is a private, nonprofit foundation. Focus is on health care rights, especially needs of Medicare beneficiaries. The Web site has links to other sites that emphasize Medicare.

301

Commission on Legal Problems of the Elderly
Phone: 202-662-8690
E-mail: abaelderly@abanet.org
Web site: www.abanet.org/elderly

The commission focuses on improving legal services for the elderly, with involvement of the private bar. It deals with elderly legal issues that surround HMO's, elder abuse, guardianship, and others. You can download an advance directive. (The commission is not active in all states.)

ElderWeb
Web site: www.elderWeb.com

Considered the "grand daddy" of aging information Web sites. It offers a wide range of topics that affect older people; it's easy to use, has great links, and is a very good site to bookmark.

Families USA
Phone: 202-347-2417
Web site: www.familiesusa.org

This is a great advocacy organization in health care and long-term care. It offers an award-winning Web site filled with consumer information on Medicare, Medicaid, prescription drug costs, a legislative action center, and Web health links. Apply your caregiving experience and become an advocate.

Meals on Wheels Association of America
Phone: 703-548-8024
Web site: www.mealsonwheelsassn.org

Track down the number of the local Meals on Wheels program in your area to have meals delivered to your parents' home, or to volunteer. Or check your local phone book for Meals on Wheels.

National Academy of Elder Law Attorneys, Inc.
Phone: 520-881-4005
Web site: www.naela.com

A nonprofit association that provides information, education, networking, and assistance to those who deal with the specialized issues of legal services to the elderly and disabled. The Web site also has a function that helps you find elder law attorneys in your area.

National Association for Hispanic Elderly
Phone: 1-800-953-8553

This agency provides information and referral services for elderly Hispanic and low-income people. Employment counseling, training, and placement services are available. Other referrals include housing, disaster relief, and income tax help.

National Association for Home Care
Phone: 202-547-7424
Web site: www.nahc.org

This nonprofit group has an excellent Web site on home health care. Learn about all of the different services and therapies available under home care. It offers a home care and hospice locator on the site. It also offers a guide on how to choose a home care provider.

National Caucus and Center on Black Aged
Phone: 202-637-8400
Web site: www.ncba-blackaged.org

The center's mission is to improve the quality of life among aging African-Americans. It is not a service provider; however, it offers programs in job opportunities, health care, housing options, and long-term care.

National Center for Home Equity Conversion
Phone: 651-222-6775
Web site: www.reverse.org

A twenty-first-century Web site devoted to the consumer. Click on "Calculator" and get an instant estimate of your home equity. Review the sources in your state for reverse equity home mortgages. Learn all you could possibly want to know about reverse mortgages before you make any decisions.

National Consumers League
Phone: 202-835-3323
E-mail: info@nclnet.org
Web site: www.nclnet.org

A private, nonprofit group advertised as the oldest consumer's group in the United States. It represents consumers on all workplace and marketplace issues. One click gives you access to information on telemarketing and Internet fraud, or drug interactions.

National Council of Senior Citizens
Phone: 1-888-373-6467
E-mail: membership@ncscerc.org
Web site: www.ncscinc.org

This organization works to improve the lives of elderly people. It is a self-described activist agency representing older Americans, with over 2,000 affiliate councils. Members can call 301-578-8938 for the Nursing Home Information Service.

National Council on the Aging
Phone: 202-479-1200
Web site: www.ncoa.org

An organization of agencies and professionals whose mission is to: "… help community organizations to enhance the lives of older adults." Click on "Aging Issues," then on "Caregiving" for information.

National Safety Council

Phone: 630-775-7615

Web site: www.nsc.org

This council stresses highway safety. Call for pamphlets and publications. On the Web site click on "Defensive Driving Training," then on "Defensive Driver Courses" to find a local site that offers the course "Coaching the Mature Driver."

National Shared Housing Resource Center

Phone: 507-433-8832

E-mail: sayoung@smig.net

Web site: www.nationalsharedhousing.org

This is a nonprofit national clearinghouse for information on shared housing. On the Web site you can click on "Directory," then choose a state and get the name, address, and phone number of a program, as well as a thumbnail description.

The National Women's Health Information Center

Office of Women's Health, DHHS

Phone: 1-800-994-9662

Web site: www.4women.gov

A Web site with a focus on women's issues. Use the "Search" box by typing in "aging," "caregiver," or "elder care" for a multitude of excellent direct links. Resource information is available on Alzheimer's, empowering caregivers and working women, and elder care.

Older Women's League (OWL)

Phone: 1-800-825-3695

E-mail: owlinfo@owl-national.org

A nonprofit, 20-year-old organization that focuses on issues of women as they age, particularly women 40 and older. There are 73 chapters nationwide. It produces an annual "Mother's Day Report"—the 2000 issue highlights prescription drug coverage legislation.

SeniorLaw

Web site: www.seniorlaw.com

Excellent one-stop source for all legal matters affecting older people. It has great links and information and its very current.

Visiting Nurses Association (VNA) of America

Phone: 1-800-426-2547

Web site: www.vnaa.org

There are over 500 VNAs throughout the country providing skilled nursing, hospice, home health aides, homemakers, nutrition advice, and personal assistance. Find a VNA near you and ask if your parents are eligible for home health care.

Books

Appleton, Michael, et al. *At Home with Terminal Illness: A Family Guidebook to Hospice in the Home*. Prentice Hall, 1994.

Beresford, Larry. *The Hospice Handbook*. Little Brown, 1993.

Byock, Ira. *Dying Well*. Putnam/Riverhead, 1997.

Carter, Rosalynn. *Helping Yourself Help Others*. Times Books, 1995.

Cosgrove, Melba, et al. *How to Survive the Loss of a Love*. Prelude, 1991.

Haman, Edward A. *How to Write Your Own Living Will*. Sourcebooks, Inc., 1997.

Kübler-Ross, Elisabeth, M.D. *On Death and Dying*. Scribner, 1997.

Llardo, Joseph A., Ph.D. *As Parents Age*. VanderWyk & Burnham, 1998.

Mace, Nancy L., and Peter V. Rabins. *The 36-Hour Day*. Johns Hopkins University Press, 1999 (first published in 1981).

Maple, Steve. *The Complete Idiot's Guide to Wills and Estates*. Alpha Books, 1997.

McLeod, Beth Witrogen. *Caregiving, the Spiritual Journey of Love, Loss and Renewal*. John Wiley & Sons, 1999.

Myers, Edward. *When Parents Die*. Penguin, 1997.

Rob, Caroline. *The Caregiver's Guide*. Houghton Mifflin Company, 1991.

Rottenberg, Dan. *The Inheritor's Handbook*. Simon & Schuster, 1999.

Secunda, Victoria. *Losing Your Parent*. Hyperion, 2000.

National List of State Units on Aging

Alabama

Commission on Aging
P.O. Box 301851
770 Washington Ave., Ste. 470
Montgomery, AL 36130-1851

Contact: Melissa Mauser Galvin,
Executive Director
Phone: 334-242-5743 or 1-800-
243-5463
Fax: 334-242-5594
E-mail: mgalvin@coa.state.al.us

Alaska

Division of Senior Services
Department of Administration
P.O. Box 110209
Juneau, AK 99811-0209

Contact: Jane Demmert, Executive
Director
Phone: 907-465-4879
Fax: 907-465-4716
E-mail: Jane_Demmert@
admin.state.ak.us

Arizona

Aging and Adult Administration
Department of Economic Security
1789 W. Jefferson, #950A
Phoenix, AZ 85007

Contact: Henry Blanco, Program
Administrator
Phone: 602-542-4446
Fax: 602-542-6575
E-mail: hblanco@mail.de.state.az.us

Arkansas

Division of Aging and Adult Services
Arkansas Department of Human
Services
P.O. Box 1437, Slot 1412
7th & Main Sts.
Little Rock, AR 72203

Contact: Herb Sanderson, Director
Phone: 501-682-2441
Fax: 501-682-8155
E-mail: herb.sanderson@mail.state.ar.us

California

Department of Aging
1600 K St.
Sacramento, CA 95814

Contact: Lynda Terry, Director
Phone: 916-322-5290
Fax: 916-324-1903
E-mail: lynda.terry@
aging.state.ca.us

Colorado

Division of Aging and Adult Services
Department of Human Services
1575 Sherman St.
Ground Fl.
Denver, CO 80203-1714

Contact: Rita Barreras, Director
Phone: 303-866-2800
Fax: 303-620-4189
E-mail: rita.barreras@state.co.us

Connecticut

Elderly Services Division
Department of Social Services
25 Sigourney St.
Hartford, CT 06106

Contact: Christine Lewis, Director
Phone: 860-424-5277
Fax: 860-424-4966
E-mail: christine.lewis@
po.state.ct.us

Delaware

Division of Services for Aging and Adults with Physical Disabilities
Department of Health and Social Services
1901 N. DuPont Hwy.
New Castle, DE 19720

Contact: Eleanor Cain, Director
Phone: 302-577-4791
Fax: 302-577-4793
E-mail: ecain@state.de.us

District of Columbia

Office on Aging
One Judiciary Square
441 4th St., N.W., 9th Fl.
Washington, DC 20001

Contact: E. Veronica Pace, Executive Director
Phone 202-724-5622
Fax: 202-724-4979

Florida

Department of Elder Affairs
Bldg. B, Ste. 152
4040 Esplanade Way
Tallahassee, FL 32399

Contact: Gema Hernandez, Secretary
Phone: 850-414-2000
Fax: 850-414-2004
E-mail: hernandezg@elderaffairs.org

Georgia

Division of Aging Services
#2 Peachtree St., N.W., #36-385
Atlanta, GA 30303

Contact: Jeffrey Minor, Director

Phone: 404-657-5258
Fax: 404-657-5285
E-mail: jaminor@dhr.state.ga.us

Guam

Division of Senior Citizens
Department of Public Health and
Social Services
Government of Guam
P.O. Box 2816
Hagaina, Guam 96932

Contact: Arthur U. San Agustin,
MHR Administrator
Phone: 011-671-475-0263
Fax: 671-477-2930
E-mail: arthursa@mail.gov.gu

Hawaii

Executive Office on Aging
No. 1 Capitol District
250 S. Hotel St., Ste 109
Honolulu, HI 96813-2831

Contact: Marilyn Seely, Director
Phone: 808-586-0100
Fax: 808-586-0185
E-mail: mrseely@health.state.hi.us

Idaho

Commission on Aging
3380 Americana Terrace, Ste. 120
P.O. Box 83720
Boise, ID 83720-0007

Contact: Lupe Wissel, Director
Phone: 208-334-2423
Fax: 208-334-3033
E-mail: lwissel@icoa.state.id.us

Illinois

Department on Aging
421 E. Capitol Ave.
Springfield, IL 62701

Contact: Margo E. Schreiber, Director
Phone: 217-785-2870
Fax: 217-785-4477
E-mail: mschreib@age084r1.state.il.us

Indiana

Bureau of Aging/In-Home Services
402 W. Washington St.
P.O. Box 7083
Indianapolis, IN 46207-7083

Contact: Geneva Shedd, Director
Phone: 317-232-7020
Fax: 317-232-7867
E-mail: gshedd@fssa.state.in.us

Iowa

Department of Elder Affairs
Clemens Bldg., 3rd Fl.
200 Tenth St.
Des Moines, IA 50309-3609

Contact: Judith Anne Conlin, Director
Phone: 515-281-5187
Fax: 515-281-4036
E-mail: judith.conlin@dea.state.ia.us

Kansas

Department on Aging
New England Bldg.
503 S. Kansas
Topeka, KS 66603-3404

Contact: Connie Hubbell, Secretary
Phone: 785-296-5222
Fax: 785-296-0256
E-mail: ConnieH@
aging.wpo.state.ks.us

Kentucky

Office of Aging Services
Cabinet for Health Services
275 E. Main St., 5 West
Frankfort, KY 40621

Contact: Jerry Whitley, Executive
Director
Phone: 502-564-6930
Fax: 502-564-4595
E-mail: jerry.whitley@
mail.state.ky.us

Louisiana

Office of Elderly Affairs
Elderly Protective Services
P.O. Box 80374
412 N. 4th St.
Baton Rouge, LA 70898-0374

Contact: Paul Arceneaux, Director
Phone: 225-342-9722
Fax: 225-342-7144

Maine

**Bureau of Elder and Adult
Services**
Department of Human Services
#11 State House Station
Augusta, ME 04333-0011

Contact: Christine Gianopoulos,
Director
Phone: 207-624-5335
Fax: 207-624-5361
E-mail: christine.gianopoulos@
state.me.us

Maryland

Department of Aging
State Office Bldg., Rm. 1007
301 W. Preston St.
Baltimore, MD 21201

Contact: Sue Ward, Secretary
Phone: 410-767-1100
Fax: 410-333-7943
E-mail: sfw@mail.ooa.state.md.us

Massachusetts

Executive Office of Elder Affairs
1 Ashburton Place, 5th Fl.
Boston, MA 02108

Contact: Lillian Glickman, Secretary
Phone: 617-727-7750
Fax: 617-727-6944
E-mail: lillian.glickman@state.ma.us

Michigan

Office of Services to the Aging
P.O. Box 30676
Lansing, MI 48909-8176

Contact: Lynn Alexander, Director
Phone: 517-373-8230
Fax: 517-373-4092
E-mail: lynn_alexander@state.mi.us

Minnesota

Board on Aging
444 Lafayette Rd.
St. Paul, MN 55155-3843

Contact: Jim Varpness, Executive
Director
Phone: 651-296-2770
Fax: 651-297-7855
E-mail: jim.varpness@state.mn.us

Mississippi

Council on Aging
Division of Aging and Adult Services
750 N. State St.
Jackson, MS 39202

Contact: Fran Bridges, Director
Phone: 601-359-4925
Fax: 601-359-4370
E-mail: fbridges@mdhs.state.ms.us

Missouri

Division of Aging
Department of Social Services
P.O. Box 1337
615 Howerton Ct.
Jefferson City, MO 65102-1337

Contact: Richard Dunn, Director
Phone: 573-751-3082
Fax: 573-751-8687
E-mail: arouth@mail.state.mo.us

Montana

Senior Long-Term Care Division
111 Sanders St.
P.O. Box 4210
Helena, MT 59604

Contact: Charles Rehbein,
Coordinator
Phone: 406-444-7788
Fax: 406-444-7743
E-mail: crehbein@state.mt.us

Nebraska

Division of Aging Services
Department of Health and Human
Services
P.O. Box 95044
301 Centennial Mall-South
Lincoln, NE 68509

Contact: Mark Intermill, Administrator
Phone: 402-471-2307
Fax: 402-471-4619
E-mail: mark.intermill@hhss.state.ne.us

Nevada

Division for Aging Services
Department of Human Resources
3416 Goni Rd., Bldg. D-132
Carson City, NV 89706

Contact: Mary Liveratti, Administrator
Phone: 775-687-4210
Fax: 775-687-4264
E-mail: dascc@govmail.state.nv.us

New Hampshire

**Division of Elderly and Adult
Services**
State Office Park South
Brown Bldg.
129 Pleasant St.
Concord, NH 03301-3857

Contact: Catherine Keane, Director
Phone: 603-271-4394
Fax: 603-271-4643
E-mail: ckeane@dhhs.state.nh.us

New Jersey

Division of Senior Affairs
Department of Health & Senior
Services
P.O. Box 807
Trenton, NJ 08625-0807

Contact: Eileen Bonilla O'Connor,
Acting Assistant Commissioner
Phone: 609-588-3141
Fax: 609-588-3317
E-mail: rreader@doh.state.nj.us

New Mexico

State Agency on Aging
La Villa Rivera Bldg.
228 E. Palace Ave., Ground Fl.
Santa Fe, NM 87501

Contact: Michelle Lujan-Grisham, Director
Phone: 505-827-7640
Fax: 505-827-7649
E-mail: michelle.grisham@state.nm.us

New York

Office for the Aging
2 Empire State Plaza
Albany, NY 12223-1251
Contact: Walter Hoefer, Director

Phone: 518-474-5731
Fax: 518-474-1398
E-mail: walter.hoefer@ofa.state.ny.us

North Carolina

Division of Aging
2101 Mail Service Center
693 Palmer Dr.
Raleigh, NC 27626-0531

Contact: Karen Gottovi, Director
Phone: 919-733-3983
Fax: 919-733-0443
E-mail: karen.gottovi@ncmail.net

North Dakota

Aging Services Division
Department of Human Services
600 S. 2nd St., Ste. 1C
Bismarck, ND 58504

Contact: Linda Wright, Director
Phone: 701-328-8910

Fax: 701-328-8989
E-mail: sowril@state.nd.us

Ohio

Department of Aging
50 W. Broad St., 9th Fl.
Columbus, OH 43215-5928

Contact: Joan W. Lawrence, Director
Phone: 614-466-5500
Fax: 614-995-1049
E-mail: jlawrence@age.state.oh.us

Oklahoma

Aging Services Division
Department of Human Services
P.O. Box 25352
312 N.E. 28th St.
Oklahoma City, OK 73105

Contact: Roy Keen, Division Administrator
Phone: 405-521-2327
Fax: 405-521-2086
E-mail: roy.keen@okdhs.org

Oregon

Senior and Disabled Services Division
500 Summer St., N.E., 2nd Fl.
Salem, OR 97310-1015

Contact: Roger Auerbach, Administrator
Phone: 503-945-5811
Fax: 503-373-7823
E-mail: roger.auerbach@state.or.us

Pennsylvania

Department of Aging
Forum Place
555 Walnut St., 5th Fl.
Harrisburg, PA 17101-1919

Contact: Richard Browdie, Secretary
Phone: 717-783-1550
Fax: 717-772-3382
E-mail: rbrowdie@pa.state.us

Puerto Rico

Governor's Office for Elderly Affairs
P.O. Box 50063
Old San Juan Station
San Juan, PR 00902

Contact: Ruby Rodriquez, Executive Director
Phone: 787-721-5710
Fax: 787-721-6510
E-mail: rrodrigu@ogave.prstar.net

Rhode Island

Department of Elderly Affairs
160 Pine St.
Providence, RI 02903-3708

Contact: Barbara Rayner, Director
Phone: 401-222-2858
Fax: 401-222-1490
E-mail: smtp:barbara@dea.state.ri.us

American-Samoa

Territorial Administration on Aging
American Samoa Government
Pago Pago, American Samoa 96799

Contact: Pc Lualemaga E. Faoa, Director
Phone: 011-684-633-1251-1252
Fax: 684-633-2533

South Carolina

Department of Health and Human Services
P.O. Box 8206
1801 Main St.
Columbia, SC 29202-8206

Contact: Elizabeth M. Fuller, Deputy Director
Phone: 803-898-2501
Fax: 803-898-4515
E-mail: fullerb@dhhs.state.sc.us

South Dakota

Office of Adult Services and Aging
700 Governors Dr.
Pierre, SD 57501

Contact: Gail Ferris, Administrator
Phone: 605-773-3656
Fax: 605-773-4855
E-mail: gailf@dss.state.sd.us

Tennessee

Commission on Aging
Andrew Jackson Bldg., 9th Fl.
500 Deaderick St.
Nashville, TN 37243-0860

Contact: James Whaley, Executive Director
Phone: 615-741-2056
Fax: 615-741-3309
E-mail: jwhaley2@mail.state.tn.us

Texas

Department on Aging
4900 N. Lamar, 4th Fl.
Austin, TX 78751-2316

Contact: Mary Sapp, Executive
Director
Phone: 512-424-6840
Fax: 512-424-6890
E-mail: mary@tdoa.state.tx.us

Utah

**Division of Aging and Adult
Services**
Department of Social Services
P.O. Box 45500
120 N.–200 W.
Salt Lake City, UT 84145-0500

Contact: Helen Goddard, Director
Phone: 801-538-3910
Fax: 801-538-4395
E-mail: HSADM2.hgoddard@
state.ut.us

Vermont

Aging and Disabilities
103 S. Main St.
Waterbury, VT 05671-2301

Contact: Patrick Flood,
Commissioner
Phone: 802-241-2400
Fax: 802-241-2325
E-mail: patrick@dad.state.vt.us

Virginia

Department for the Aging
1600 Forest Ave.
Preston Bldg., Ste. 102
Richmond, VA 23229

Contact: Ann McGee, Commissioner
Phone: 804-662-9333
Fax: 804-662-9354
E-mail: amcgee@vdh.state.va.us

Virgin Islands

Senior Citizen Affairs
Department of Human Services
#19 Estate Diamond Fredericksted
St. Croix, VI 00840

Contact: Bernice Hall, Administrator
Phone: 340-692-5950
Fax: 340-692-2062

Washington

**Aging and Adult Services
Administration**
Department of Social and Health
Services
P.O. Box 45050
Olympia, WA 98504-5050

Contact: Kathy Leitch, Acting Assistant
Secretary
Phone: 360-902-7797
Fax: 360-902-7848
E-mail: leitckj@dshs.wa.gov

West Virginia

**West Virginia Bureau of Senior
Services**
1900 Kanawha Blvd, E.
Holly Grove-Bldg. 10
Charleston, WV 25305-0160

Contact: Gaylene A. Miller,
Commissioner
Phone: 304-558-5609
Fax: 304-558-5609
E-mail: gmiller@boss.state.wv.us

Wisconsin

Bureau of Aging and Long Term Care Resources
Department of Health and Family Services
One W. Wilson St.
P.O. Box 7851
Madison, WI 53707-7851

Contact: Donna McDowell, Director
Phone: 608-266-2536
Fax: 608-267-3203
E-mail: mcdowdb@dhfs.state.wi.us

Wyoming

Department of Health, Division on Aging
Hathaway Bldg., Rm. 139
Cheyenne, WY 82002-0710

Contact: Daniel G. Stackis, Administrator
Phone: 307-777-7986 or 1-800-442-2766
Fax: 307-777-5340
E-mail: wmilto@missc.state.wy.us

Dr. Rhodes' Nursing Home Navigator

Researching a good nursing home (skilled nursing facility) is no small task, especially if you're doing the research during a medical crisis. My navigational guide should help you get a solid start—but it's not meant to be the only tool you use. The ombudsman, too, can be very helpful to you. This person's name and phone number are posted in the lobby of the nursing home.

Part 1 identifies questions you can ask over the phone to narrow your search. Ask to speak to the Admissions Director. Part 2 centers on Nursing Home Survey and Inspection Reports. It guides you on how to get the reports, what to look for, and how to
interpret the findings. Part 3 gives you a list of things to look for when you visit the facility. Throughout the guide, you're given tips to help you better understand why you're asking these questions. Feel free to make copies of this guide for each facility you research.

Part 1: Narrowing Your Search

Name of facility:

_____

Address and phone number:

_____

_____

Medicare certified?_____ Bed capacity _____ No. filled _____ (Note: If it has a large vacancy rate, ask why. If not, ask if there is a wait.)

Special units (for example, rehab, Alzheimer's)

_____

Who doesn't it accept? (for example, residents who are ventilator-dependent, oxygen-dependent, on dialysis, have a tracheostomy)

_____

Is this a for-profit facility? _____ Who owns it?

_____

Is it part of a chain?

_____

Is this a nonprofit facility? _____ Affiliation?

_____

Does it have a hospital affiliation?

_____

What is the cost?

_____

Does your parent qualify for Medicaid? What will Medicare cover? What will any other insurance your parent has cover?

_____

Is there a volunteer program? Please describe:

_____

_____

Staffing Questions:

What kind of a background check does it conduct on staff?

_____

What is your turnover rate? _____ (How often staff quit and are replaced) What are you doing to reduce it?

_____

_____

How many physical therapists are on staff? _____ Employee or contracted?

_____

How many occupational therapists? _____ Employee or contracted?

_____

How many speech therapists? _____ Employee or contracted? _____

Tip: These therapists assist people recovering from strokes and help others from deteriorating. A full-time employee is more likely to offer continuity of care for your parent than someone who is contracted through an agency.

How many hours of training do nurse's aides receive per year? _____

Have nurse's aides received training in abuse prevention? _____

How many nurse's aides per resident? _____

How many minutes per day do nurse's aides spend on directly caring for a resident? _____

Tip: Residents do better when nurse's aides spend at least 2 hours per day per resident. Look for homes closer to reaching this benchmark. The federal minimum standard, however, is lower than this. So you may find many homes that don't reach this benchmark.

What is the state's minimum staffing level for nurse's aides per resident? _____
How much does the home exceed this minimum?

_____

How many nurse's aides per resident during morning shift: _____ Afternoon shift: _____ Evening shift: _____ Weekends: _____

Tip: Look at how much these ratios change during shifts. Evening shifts may be lower because residents are sleeping. Watch for any major cutbacks during weekends. The more staff per resident the better. When you compare homes, look for the facility with more staff and with lower staff turnover rates. Studies show that nonprofit homes significantly employ more staff to care for residents than do for-profits.

How many registered nurses does it employ? _____

Are these nurses full-time employees or are they employed through a temp agency?

_____

How many minutes per day do registered nurses spend per resident? _____

If your parent has a medical condition requiring more time, how will the home accommodate his or her special needs?

_____

_____

Tips: The more registered nurses (RNs), the better. If the home employs temp agency RNs, then nurse's aides aren't as likely to receive consistent supervision. Permanent employees are better. Also, if the facility accepts residents with complex needs like people with chronic lung disease, people on dialysis, or people dependent on oxygen or ventilators, look for the facility to hire more registered nurses.

Part 2: Nursing Home Deficiency and Survey Reports

Every nursing home is inspected by state and federal agencies. Each agency issues a report on any deficiencies it finds at the facility. The federal government reports the results of these reports on the Internet. Go to www.medicare.gov and click on Nursing Home Compare. This should be part of your research.

Even very good homes will have a few deficiencies. You want to look at what those deficiencies are and how serious—was someone hurt or were the residents placed in jeopardy because of the deficiency? When doing your research, follow these steps:

- Look up the home on Nursing Home Compare and see if the home has had serious deficiencies and a pattern of them. You'll find this on the Internet at www.medicare.gov.

- Ask for the name of the facility's ombudsman and how to contact him or her. This should be posted on the nursing home's bulletin board in the lobby. Give the ombudsman a call for help in sorting through your research.

    Ombudsman's name: _____

    Phone: _____

- Ask for a copy of the home's most recent survey report.

Here are my top 10 red flags you should look for in the report. Has the home been cited in any of the following areas:

- **Care assessments.** Every resident must have a care plan, which means the resident has been assessed by an interdisciplinary team.

- **Physical restraints.** Residents should not be physically restrained in beds or chairs in which they can't get out; nor should they be chemically restrained (sedated to keep them immobile).

- **Bladder treatment.** For incontinent residents, not getting proper care changing adult briefs or bedding.

- **Hydration.** Residents not getting enough fluids.

- **Catheter use.** For incontinent residents, improper catheter care or catheter being used when it's not necessary.

- **Infection control.** Residents exposed to infections because of poor sanitation or staff not following infection control practices.

- **Pressure (bed) sores.** Open sores usually caused by lack of turning patients and poor skin care.

- **Unnecessary drugs.** Residents being given drugs they don't need.

- **Medication errors.** Mistakes in giving residents the wrong drug, wrong combination of drugs, or wrong dosage.
- **Malnutrition incidence.** Residents found to be malnourished. This is some times due to a lack of staff to take the time to help feed patients or encourage them to eat.

If you see these types of deficiencies on the report, look at how severe the deficiency was: Did it cause actual harm or place residents in jeopardy? Did the inspectors identify this as a pattern or was it a one-time occurrence. The report spells this out.

Fall reports: Ask the administrator to see the facility's annual report on incidents of falls. A high fall rate may indicate inadequate staffing. The ombudsman should be able to help you determine if the fall rate is high or not.

Ban on admissions: Ask the administrator if the home has ever had a ban on admissions. Ask when, what for, and how it was corrected. Also ask the ombudsman to give you the full story. When state or federal inspectors find very severe problems at a home, they ban the home from admitting any new residents.

Complaints: Usually, state departments of health and local health departments investigate complaints made against nursing homes. Ask the ombudsman to tell you if this home has an unusual number of complaints made against it and how severe. The ombudsman can also tell you whom to contact to receive public complaint information.

If you have further questions, ask the ombudsman to help you interpret the report, and also ask the nursing home administrator to clarify anything you don't under-stand.

Part 3: Walking Through the Facility

Now it's time to trust your instincts and your senses. Don't just stay in a fancy lobby or administrator's office when you visit the facility. (If you visit a resident's room, be sure to get permission from the resident before you enter.) Here are some of the things you should look for, with space to jot down your observations:

- Does it feel like home? Are there personal effects in the rooms?

- Are staff interacting in a friendly manner with each other and the residents?

- Is the home free of odors? Is it clean? Well lit?

- Is the temperature comfortable? Stop by a few rooms to see. (Many older folks like their rooms warmer than what you might like—is the room too cold?)

- Are residents well groomed? Are they dressed appropriately for the time of day?

  _____

- Where are the residents? In halls? In group activity rooms? In their rooms appearing isolated?

  _____

- Is there a wandering alert system?

  _____

- Is there an activity calendar? Are there pictures on the bulletin boards showing recent activities? Are the activities interesting and varied?

  _____

- Are there active volunteers helping out?

  _____

- Are lavatories clean?

  _____

- Are food trays left sitting out—and do you see a lot of leftover food on the trays?

  _____

- Are call buttons left unanswered for long periods of time?

  _____

- Ask to see the menus. Does the food sound appetizing? Ask about the qualifications of the person who oversees the menus. Taste the food, if possible.

  _____

- Are there any safety hazards?

  _____

- Does the equipment look up to date and in good condition?

  _____

- Is the outdoor area secure so that no one can wander off into an unsafe area?

  _____

- Go to the dining room—are residents enjoying themselves? Is it pleasant? Is staff interacting with the residents?

  _____

- Are bed linens and towels cleaned daily? Ask what the laundry department does to prevent bed sores? (Poorly cleaned, starchy sheets and certain detergents can cause skin breakdown.)

  _____

- Are soiled linens piled up in the hallways or in residents' rooms?

  _____

- Are showers clean? Look for safety devices to prevent falls.

  _____

- Is there fresh water on nightstands easily accessible for residents?

  _____

Additional Notes:

_____

_____

_____

_____

_____

_____

Reprint permission granted for personal use only.

Nursing Home Bill of Rights

RESIDENTS' RIGHTS IN NURSING HOMES
Consumer Information Sheet

If you are a resident or have a loved one in a nursing home, this information highlights your rights. **Residents' rights** are part of the federal Nursing Home Reform Law enacted in 1987 in the Social Security Act. The law requires nursing homes to "promote and protect the rights of each resident" and places a strong emphasis on individual dignity and self-determination. Nursing homes must meet residents' rights requirements if they participate in Medicare or Medicaid. The following is an overview of the ways that the law protects residents' rights.

Quality of Life

The Nursing Home Reform Law requires each nursing home to "care for its residents in such a manner and in such an environment as will promote maintenance or enhancement of the quality of life of each resident." This requirement emphasizes dignity, choice, and self-determination for residents.

Providing Services and Activities

Each nursing home is required to "provide services and activities to attain or maintain the highest practicable physical, mental, and psychosocial well-being of each resident in accordance with a written plan of care which ... is initially prepared, with participation to the extent practicable of the resident, the resident's family, or legal representative." This means that a resident should not decline in health or well-being as a result of the way a nursing facility provides care.

Specific Rights

The Nursing Home Reform Law legally protects the following rights for nursing home residents:

The Right to Be Fully Informed, including the right to:
- Be informed of all services available as well as the charge for each service;
- Have a copy of the nursing home's rules and regulations, including a written copy of resident rights;
- Be informed of the address and telephone number of the State Ombudsman, State survey agency office, and other advocacy groups;
- See the State survey reports of the nursing home and the home's plan of correction;
- Be notified in advance of any plans to change their room or roommate;
- Daily communication in the resident's language, for example, Spanish;
- Assistance if they have a sensory impairment.

The Right to Participate in Their Own Care, including the right to:
- Receive adequate and appropriate care;
- Be informed of any changes in their medical condition;
- Participate in their assessment, care-planning, treatment, and discharge;
- Refuse medication and treatment;
- Refuse chemical and physical restraints;
- Review their medical record.

The Right to Make Independent Choices, including the right to:
- Make independent personal decisions, such as what to wear and how to spend free time;
- Reasonable accommodation of their needs and preferences by the nursing home;
- Choose their own physician;
- Participate in community activities, both inside and outside the nursing home;
- Organize and participate in a Resident Council or other resident advisory group.

The Right to Privacy and Confidentiality, including the right to:
- Private and unrestricted communication with any person of their choice;
- Privacy in treatment and in the care of their personal needs;
- Confidentiality regarding their medical, personal, or financial affairs.

©1999. National Citizens' Coalition for Nursing Home Reform, 1424 16th Street, NW, Suite 202, Washington, D.C. 20036. Tel. 202-332-2275, Fax 202-332-2949, e-mail: nccnhr@nccnhr.org, Web site: www.nccnhr.org

The Right to Dignity, Respect, and Freedom, including the right to:

- Be treated with the fullest measure of consideration, respect, and dignity;
- Be free from mental and physical abuse, corporal punishment, involuntary seclusion, and physical and chemical restraints;
- Self-determination.

The Right to Security of Possessions, including:

- Manage their own financial affairs;
- File a complaint with the State survey and certification agency for abuse, neglect, or misappropriation of their property if the nursing home is handling their financial affairs;
- Be free from charge for services covered by Medicaid or Medicare.

Rights During Transfers and Discharges, including:

- Remain in the nursing facility unless a transfer or discharge:
  (a) is necessary to meet the resident's welfare;
  (b) is appropriate because the resident's health has improved and the resident no longer requires nursing home care;
  (c) is needed to protect the health and safety of other residents or staff; or
  (d) is required because the resident has failed, after reasonable notice, to pay the facility charge for an item or service provided at the resident's request;
- Receive thirty-day notice of transfer or discharge. The notice must include the reason for transfer or discharge, the effective date, the location to which the resident is transferred or discharged, a statement of the right to appeal, and the name, address, and telephone number of the state long-term care ombudsman;
- A safe transfer or discharge through sufficient preparation by the nursing home.

The Right to Complain, including the right to:

- Present grievances to the staff of the nursing home, or to any other person, without fear of reprisal;
- Prompt efforts by the nursing home to resolve grievances;
- Complain to the survey agency and ombudsman program.

The Right to Visits, including the right to:

- Immediate access by a resident's personal physician and representatives from the state survey agency and ombudsman programs;
- Immediate access by their relatives and for others "subject to reasonable restriction" with the resident's permission;
- Reasonable visits by organizations or individuals providing health, social, legal, or other services.

Advocates for Residents Rights

The Long Term Care Ombudsman Program is required by federal law to promote and protect the rights of residents of nursing homes and related facilities, such as board and care homes. Contact your local or state ombudsman for information and assistance with making sure that resident rights are respected. Many states also have citizen advocacy groups that champion resident rights. Obtain contact information for your state or local ombudsman and citizen advocacy groups by contacting the National Citizens' Coalition for Nursing Home Reform at 202-332-2275, e-mail: nccnhr@nccnhr.org, Web site: www.nccnhr.org.

If you are interested in learning more, the National Citizens' Coalition for Nursing Home Reform (NCCNHR) has several publications that may be of interest. Call 202-332-2275 for a publication list or visit the Web site at http://www.nccnhr.org.

➢ **Nursing Homes: Getting Good Care There -- Consumer Book,** Cost: $14.95

➢ **Avoiding Physical Restraint Use - consumer booklet,** Cost: $7.50

➢ **Avoiding Drugs Used as Chemical Restraints -- consumer booklet,** Cost: $7.50

Order both (1 of each) Restraint booklets for $14

➢ **Using Resident Assessment and Care Planning: An Advocacy Tool for Residents and their Advocates,** Cost: $12

Prices listed do not include shipping and handling.

Websites

Dr. Rhodes' Government Picks for Caring for Your Parent

For hot links to all sites referenced here and throughout this book, go to www. lindarhodes.com.

Access America for Seniors
www.seniors.gov

A one-stop site featuring government and agency services for seniors.

Administration on Aging
www.aoa.gov

This federal agency acts as hub of all government aging services and provides a network of state and area agencies on aging. The Web site is chock full of information and links to other government sites.

Eldercare Locator
1-800-677-1116
www.eldercare.gov

Directs you to local and regional agencies for senior services. Connects you to your local area agency on aging. A great resource.

Healthfinder
www.healthfinder.gov

A gateway to consumer health and human services info from the U.S. Department of Health and Human Services. The Web site offers a directory of services and links to agencies and databases. Great site and easy to use.

Housing and Urban Development (HUD)
1-888-569-4287
www.hud.gov

This federal agency runs low-income housing for seniors as well as other services.

Medicare Hotline
1-800-638-6833
www.medicare.gov

Offers a complete guide on Medicare, including Nursing Home Compare—which posts national survey reports on all homes and allows you to compare them—and a comparison guide on managed care plans.

National Institutes of Health

www.nih.gov

A major hub site for health information via Medline. Hosts National Institutes of Aging, Mental Health, and Cancer. Find clinical trials and reviews of 9,000 prescription and over-the-counter drugs.

Social Security Administration (SSA)

1-800-772-1213

www.ssa.gov

This federal agency runs Social Security retirement, survivor's benefits, disability insurance, and Supplemental Security Income (SSI). The Web site answers most questions. Easy to use.

Veterans Administration (VA)

1-800-827-1000

www.va.gov

The federal VA system offers benefits to veterans. The Web site offers a full range of benefits, eligibility and contact info, and medical services.

Dr. Rhodes' Basic Three for Caring for Aging Parents

American Association of Retired Persons (AARP)

1-800-424-3410

www.aarp.org

The largest aging consumer group in the country. Great information.

Elderweb

www.elderweb.com

The "grand daddy" of aging information Web sites, resources, and news.

National Council on Aging "Benefits Check-Up"

www.benefitscheckup.org

Fill out a simple questionnaire and immediately find out if your parent qualifies for benefits and prescription discounts. Provides forms and contact data.

Senior Law

www.seniorlaw.com

An excellent source on a wide range of legal needs and issues of seniors.

Dr. Rhodes' Best Caregiving Web Sites for Caring for Aging Parents

www.agenet.com

Commercial site: good all-around info, resource info, links, news, support group chat rooms, and products.

www.alz.org

National Alzheimer's Association: educational, resource information, excellent links, find an Alzheimer chapter near you; or call 1-800-272-3900.

www.caps4caregivers.org

Children of Aging Parents offers excellent resources for family members, links, support groups, fact sheets, and newsletters. You can also call them at 1-800-227-7294.

www.caregiver.com

This site offers a free e-mail newsletter and free articles on caregiving along with links and products. It features extremely helpful *Caregiver* magazine that you can order online.

www.caregiver.org

Family Caregiver Alliance: resource info, caregiving tips, ask an online expert, fact sheets, support group, chat rooms, and links.

www.caregiving.org

National Alliance for Caregiving: resource info, caregiving advice, reports, fact sheets, links, and news.

www.caremanager.org

National Association of Professional Geriatric Care Managers: resource info and U.S. directory of care managers you can contact.

www.healthinaging.org

The American Geriatrics Society Foundation for Health in Aging offers a free online guide for caregivers and identifies geriatricians in your area. You can also call them at 1-800-563-4916.

www.lindarhodes.com

This is a companion site to Dr. Rhodes' book *Caregiving as Your Parents Age* featuring links to nearly 100 Web sites identified in her book. You can also order her *Caregiver Kit from Linda Rhodes Caregiving*™ featured on QVC online or call 1-800-345-1212.

www.nfcacares.org

National Family Caregiver Association is a grass roots group that educates and supports families. Their site offers links, programs, services, public awareness, and advocacy.

www.seniorlaw.com

A top-flight source on a wide range of legal needs and issues affecting older people.

Index

Numbers

A

M

P–Q

T

U–V

W–X–Y–Z